The Insiders' Guide to Medical Schools 2001/2002

The Alternative
Prospectus
compiled by the
BMA Medical
Students Committee

Edited by

**Ian Urmston
Deborah Cohen
Richard Partridge**

BMJ
Books

© BMJ Books 2001
BMJ Books is an imprint of the BMJ Publishing Group

First published in 1998
by BMJ Books, BMA House, Tavistock Square,
London WC1H 9JR

www.bmjbooks.com

First edition 1998
Second edition 1999
Third edition 2000
Fourth edition 2001

British Library Cataloguing in Publication Data

A catalogue record for this book is available from the
British Library

ISBN 0-7279-1660-2

Typeset by FiSH Books, London
Printed and bound in Great Britain by MPG Books Ltd, Bodmin, Cornwall

Contents

Ian Urmston works in the Marketing Department at the British Medical Association. He is married to Sarah and they have two boys Jos and Finn.

Deborah Cohen is a fourth year medical student at Manchester Medical School.

Richard Patridge is a medical student at the nearly merged Royal Free and University College Medical School. He studied for an intercalated degree last year in medical journalism and is currently in his first clinical year.

Foreword

Welcome to the updated edition of "The Insiders' Guide to Medical Schools" – your guide to applying to medical school in the UK. Each UK medical school is featured, with the chapter being written by a medical student currently studying there. The authors of the chapters are members of the BMA's Medical Students Committee, and have attempted to tell you the reality of studying medicine at their school – the good, the bad, and the positively ugly!

This is a time of much change in undergraduate medicine – with more and more scientific and technological advances being made every day, it is no longer possible to learn "everything" at medical school. Universities are now attempting to equip students with the skills they need to access information and continue to develop professionally, long after the graduation ceremony is behind them. Whilst the core topics to be studied are determined by the General Medical Council, the way in which teaching and learning is approached differs between the individual schools – with some offering a course based mainly on self-directed problem solving, and some retaining a more traditional lecture based curriculum. Undoubtedly different people are more suited to different styles of learning, and hopefully you'll be able to use this book, in conjunction with the university prospectuses, to help you choose the kind of institution, course and location that's right for you.

Despite the big workload and increasing cost of studying to be a doctor, as medical students we are still in a very special position. We are given the opportunity to work with our patients during some of their most difficult and personal moments, and our course is a unique blend of science and humanities. Enjoy deciding how to fill in that UCAS form, and good luck!

Kate Duffield
Chair
BMA Medical Students Committee

The book is updated every year by the BMA's Medical Students Committee, which represents 12 000 medical students in the UK. If you have any suggestions for ways the *Insiders' Guide* could be improved we'd like to hear them. Send them to the editor at iurmston@bma.org.uk

Preface

Deciding to study medicine and applying to medical school is a big step. The vocational nature of the medical degree means that you are making a decision about a course of study and also your future career.

All of us who put this book together know what a nerve-wracking time it is; as current medical students it is still very fresh in all our minds. But even in the few years since we applied, pressures on applicants have increased. Higher entrance requirements, and mounting financial pressures, need to be considered but shouldn't put you off.

Through this book we hope to be able to use our hindsight to guide you through making this decision. We'll be able to answer some of your questions – the same questions we too were asking a few years ago. We'll also be able to give you some insiders' tips on the application process, medical student life, and on some of the things we have only found out ourselves since applying.

Of course choosing to study medicine is only part of the story. Choosing the right medical school for you is equally important if you want to maximise your time at university. While a book like this could never claim complete objectivity or compete with all the definitive information from all the medical schools, the strength of our *Insiders' Guide* is the fact that we are all medical students. We hope to be able to offer you a viewpoint from people who were, not so long ago, in the position you are in now. To complete the picture, there is a section on what happens after graduation.

We hope our comments are helpful, but please take them as one part of a bigger picture. Everyone – the medical schools, your teachers, your friends, your family – will be giving you advice (or even pressure). The important thing is that you make sure you are fully informed and that it is *you* who makes the ultimate decision as to whether it's to be medicine, and, if so, where you want to study.

We wish you luck in your application.

Deborah Cohen and Richard Partridge

Acknowledgements and contributors

We would like to thank all the many individuals and institutions who have provided the information and views contained in this book; it would not have been possible without their help. We would also like to thank the many BMA and BMJ staff, in particular Remi of the MSC Secretariat and Alex from BMJ Books, who have helped massively at various stages in the preparation of this book. Their support and efforts on our behalf have been invaluable and are very much appreciated. To all the contributors, both past and present, we say a big, big thank-you.

Aderonke Adeniji, Bushra Alam, Dave Allen, Dan Atkinson, Parham Azerbod, Pedram Azerbod, Kenneth Baillie, Iain Beardsell, Caroline Beck, Ian Benton, Georgina Burnham, Lucy Burr, Mobasher Butt, Jennifer Campbell, Paul Carter, Claire Castledine, Narendra Chandratre, Nazia Chaudhuri, Jennie Ciechan, Sarah Cluskey, Deborah Cohen, Mike Cordner, Lizz Corps, Emily Craft, Laurence Crutchlow, Kate Duffield, Alan Duncan, Rebecca Ebsworth, Katrina Farrell, Joseph Footit, Amy Fora, Mark Glover, Natalie Glover, Richard Graham, Emma Gray, Mark Haines, Sarah Haines, Derek Hilton, Liza Hirst, Dominic Hurford, Elspeth Isbiter, Nick Jenkins, Andrew Jinks, Nina Johns, Paul Johnstone, Ambreen Kalhoro, Baylon Kamalarajan, Karan Kapoor, Janan Katib, Janet Kerr, Aalia Khan, Anjum Khan, Michelle Kidd, Elizabeth Kingston, Natasha Lelli, Rachel Lindley, Kiera Lindsay, Nicola Littlewood, Nicholas Love, John Loy, Katharine MacDowall, Ruth MacPherson, Edel McAuley, Kathy McCann, Jim McCaul, Claire McCombie, Remy McConvey, Victoria McCormack, Brigit McGuigan, Adele McKenna, Derek McLaughlan, Tony Matheson, Kristian Mears, Omer Moghraby, Michael Moneypenny, Aruna Muna-Singhe, Clodagh Murphy, Molin Navamani, Helen Neary, Seamus Phillips, Fenella Powell, Saul Rajak, Leeanne Ramdin, Alan Robertson, Jonathon Rohrer, Anusa Sabanathan, Rameen Shakur, Zoe Silverstone, Rebecca Smith, Sarah Snowden, Alistair Steel, Sian Stephens, James Stoddart, Ximena Thomas, Ian Thompson, Louise Turner, Michael Urdang, Salima Wahab, Katie Ward, Anne-Marie Wilcox, Michael Williams, Matt Williams-Gray, James Wood, Martin Wood, and Alistair Woodman, Chris Zollo.

With apologies to any students we might have accidentally missed out.

Using this book

This book gives valuable information and views about studying medicine in the UK. It will help any student considering medicine as a career option as well as those of you who already know that you want to become a doctor. The strength of this book is that it has been compiled by medical students themselves. It will give you the kind of information and opinions that are not always in medical school prospectuses or in the UCAS handbooks.

Now, it won't surprise you that student life differs radically from one university to the next, but it might surprise you that each medical school offers a course which, to some extent, is unique. It is important when drawing up your short list to choose only those schools with course structures and styles which suit you in towns or cities where you could be happy. Medics, more than anyone else, can give you the low-down on the distinguishing features you might want to consider.

A book like this, however, could never claim to be totally objective or definitive about all the differences and similarities between the medical schools. Take the views offered here into account and use this information alongside other materials you will have collected (for example prospectuses) as you draw up your short list of where to apply.

Remember

- Read the medical/university prospectus
- Read the alternative prospectus (if available)
- Visit the medical school (some have open days) and the town or city
- Visit the medical school website

Choosing medicine

Ask the average sixth former why he or she is applying to study medicine, and they'll probably tell you it's because they enjoy science and want to help patients. Probe a little deeper and they may mention ideas such as money, kudos, and the fact that they are expected to get good A level grades. Medicine may command a certain amount of kudos (or even sex appeal) and doctors tend to be held in high regard by the general public. Qualifying as a doctor practically guarantees you the means of earning a living (numbers entering medical school are increasing but are subject to strict control) and the pay is good. Junior doctors can get paid an annual salary of £20,000+, but they work very long and hard for it. As you work your way up the profession the pay gets better and there is sometimes scope for private income. However, if your only aim in medicine is to make stacks of dosh, to prance around in a white coat looking like a star from a TV drama, or to prove how able you are to pass exams, forget it. There are many easier ways to make a million, the work is only occasionally glamorous; application and dedication to patient care and learning are far more important attributes than the ability to continually pass difficult exams.

Doctors are respected members of any community, and a MORI poll last year showed that the public's trust in doctors is still very high. But with this respect comes responsibility and pressure. You only need to read a small selection of newspapers to see that doctors are a major focus of media attention and public interest. Not all of the resulting coverage is favourable and/or fair. Knowing that you are under constant scrutiny, and not always from people who understand clinical medicine, adds to the stresses of the job. As a doctor, you will be faced with difficult decisions involving ethical and clinical dilemmas and these situations can be very stressful. There are also many unpleasant tasks, like breaking bad news or dealing with an abusive patient or relative. You have to deal professionally with patients, and the bald truth is that they are not all lovely people. Curing patients is fulfilling and exciting – it happens regularly in some specialties – but there will be many patients you can't cure, many symptoms that can't be controlled, and many "worried well" who can't be persuaded that they are not in fact ill.

To follow particular career directions within medicine you will need to study and sit postgraduate exams. It is vital that you continue your medical education if you are to keep your skills and knowledge up to date. Junior doctors often feel overworked and undervalued, and it is not uncommon, at some stage in their career, for doctors to question whether they are in the right job at all. Several factors, such as long hours, stress and poor accommodation, can combine to make working conditions unpleasant. The British Medical Association (BMA) is the doctors' trade union and professional organisation. It has sought, in negotiation with government, to reduce the hours of work and improve doctors' terms and conditions of service. Some of the excesses you might have heard about in the media are being addressed but there are still many problems that remain unresolved. At the time of writing the BMA's Junior Doctor Committee has agreed a new pay deal for junior doctors. The Deal has removed overtime rates of pay which were less than the normal hourly rate. The new system involves paying a supplement on top of a basic salary to pay for out-of-hours work. The value of the supplement is aimed to reflect the working pattern, intensity of work and the anti-social nature of the post. Different levels of supplement apply to different posts.

The medical profession is increasingly diverse. As this diversity increases, so too do the opportunities to work less than full time or combine different areas of practice as you follow your career. Doctors working flexible hours or job-sharing are more common than in previous generations. Ethnic minorities comprise 30% of the intake to medical school, and just over 20% of the medical workforce. Sadly, it would be untrue to say that racial and sex discrimination never occur within medical schools or the health service, but the BMA and the NHS Executive are very active in promoting equal opportunities.

Many gay, lesbian and bisexual applicants are unsure how their sexuality may affect their future career. While some within the profession may hold unsympathetic views, they are an ever-decreasing minority. Be reassured that gay, lesbian and bisexual doctors are found at all grades, across all specialties. While many are happy to be open about their sexuality with colleagues, others still prefer to keep their personal lives private.

Being a medical student involves many hours in lectures, tutorials, practicals, clinics, and wards. The course is intellectually and emotionally demanding and medics are accumulating ever-increasing debts (but don't be put off by the debts alone – you'll earn more than enough to pay it off later on). Your friends studying for other degrees may have as many hours time tabled per week as you'll have per day – and you'll have to study in the evening. Medical degree courses normally last five or six years. Graduates from other, shorter courses may be in a job and earning more money than you will be when you qualify, and you may still have two more years of unpaid study left before you get a salary.

Don't be surprised if you have any doubts about studying medicine. Many potential medics will also be flirting with the idea of pharmacy, law, veterinary sciences, and other courses. Speak to some doctors – your own GP might be a start – or arrange some work experience at your local hospital. Entering medicine is not a decision to take lightly or for the wrong reasons. It's a long haul, and requires a commitment and devotion that far exceed any financial rewards. Whatever combination of reasons has made you choose medicine, remember it is a vocation. Those who enter medical school with a strong commitment to work hard and learn, and who want to serve patients, are the students most likely to find life as a doctor richly rewarding and stimulating.

Life as a medical student

In the past there was a school of thought that viewed medical students as spending their first couple of years cramming a vast amount of knowledge without ever seeing a patient, and then emerging brainwashed, unable to think and unable to communicate. Well, if this ever was the case, it is now certainly a thing of the past. Recognising some problems in medical school training, the General Medical Council (GMC) published a report in 1993 called *Tomorrow's doctors*, telling medical schools to reduce the emphasis on learning factual information and concentrate much more on developing the skills and attitudes needed to become a doctor. The report also recommended the introduction of Special Study Modules (SSMs) to give students the chance to undertake projects of their own choosing. Alongside this the GMC encouraged schools to adopt a more "problem-based" learning approach to teaching, where facts are taught within a framework of real-to-life clinical scenarios. Developing research skills and encouraging intellectual curiosity and enthusiasm for learning is now as important as knowledge.

Most schools have already changed their curricula and others are in the process of changing, so that older courses (in which science and clinical practice were taught separately) have almost completely given way to integrated curricula. In other words, instead of learning anatomy, then biochemistry, then physiology, students are more likely to learn about respiration, reproduction, diet, and metabolism. In most schools students will have some regular contact with clinicians and patients from the outset. The early years still have less clinical content and more lecture and lab teaching, but the traditional pre-clinical/clinical divide is dying. An important effect of these changes is that students need to be much more responsible for their own studies and lots of self-motivation is needed. New clinical skills labs have been introduced in many schools so that students can practise procedures and examinations on dummies. This helps build confidence before going on the wards and meeting patients.

The balance between lectures, problem-based learning, SSMs and clinical exposure will vary between medical schools and should be spelt out in each prospectus. The clinical work takes place in local teaching hospitals and district general hospitals (DGHs), which may be many miles away from the medical school. These "attachments" take you out of town, but getting away from the big city hospitals can give you the chance to be more useful and learn more. Most schools provide free accommodation within the hospitals if commuting is not practicable. Some schools will even allow overseas attachments in addition to the elective (see below).

As you would imagine, there is a fair amount of blood and gore in medicine at various stages (for example physiology practicals, post-mortems, dissection, taking blood samples – including your own, as a house officer and during surgery). Many students become used to this remarkably quickly. For others, it may take longer. It may surprise you to know that some doctors are still squeamish after many years of practice. If you are very concerned about how you might react, try to arrange some appropriate work experience at your local hospital.

You can interrupt most courses by studying for an extra "intercalated" degree. This is normally a medical science degree (BSc, BMedSci) undertaken during an extra year (or two) of study. It is commonly taken after the second or third year, and entry policies vary between schools. It is compulsory in some, actively encouraged in others while some allow it by invitation only. In some schools where it is voluntary, as many as 50% of each year group intercalate at some stage in their studies. The main consideration to be given to extending an already long course to complete an intercalated degree is the issue of financing the extra 12 months. At some schools and in some situations tuition fees for the intercalated degree year are paid for, but you will still need to finance maintenance for an extra year.

During the final years of the course there is normally a medical elective. This is a period of weeks or months when students travel to a specialist clinic or hospital attachment of their own choice. This can be in the UK, but many medics use the opportunity to go overseas and learn about medicine in the developing world, a particular disease or condition, or another system of healthcare delivery. Electives can be the high point of medical student life. Students who get organised early enough can usually find enough funding for an elective to help avoid paying for all of it themselves. Many combine the elective with some extra travel and a holiday. The length of time available for the elective(s) depends on the medical school. There is normally some sort of information held locally about where students have been in recent years which might help you decide where to go. Missionary, voluntary and charity organisations can sometimes help you find a suitable clinic or hospital to visit or academic departments at your medical school may have some pre-packaged electives with fellow institutes abroad.

The GMC puts great emphasis on skills and attitudes rather than the traditional rote learning of huge amounts of facts. Increasingly, formal lectures are out and problem-based integrated learning is in! However, there are still exams. Many medical schools examine by continuous assessment and have rearranged the finals so that they are taken over a period of time rather than all at once. This has been a sensible development and has reduced a lot of the periodic pressure. Some, however, would argue that this has only spread the pressure throughout the year; the increased number of exams can lead to exam fatigue, and at many schools "finals" are still dreaded. After finals, guess what? More exams in whatever postgraduate specialty you choose!

Being a medical student is enjoyable but hard work. It soon becomes apparent that the commitments and expectations are far greater than applicants might have expected, and also far greater than those of your friends on other degree courses. Attendance at lectures/practicals/clinical sessions can last from 9 a.m. until 5 p.m. every day and a register might be taken. Medics have to compare this with other students who might only have four hours of lectures a week! Additional time is needed for personal study and revision. Exams also demand time and energy for preparation.

Despite all these pressures, medical students have no trouble being sporty and sociable. In fact, we often excel at both. There is a wide mix of students at every medical school and every group will contain a range of public school and state school, working class and middle class, medical family and non-medical family type backgrounds. You will be able to pursue your non-course interests as well as your studies. "Work hard and play hard" is the maxim which unites medical students and the medical profession has an enviable community spirit – a "we're all in it together" attitude. Year groups are generally large (100+), and, because everyone is doing the same course, you get to know your colleagues very quickly and very well. The downside of this is that medical students sometimes have a reputation for not mixing with other students. It is also why we have a good reputation for relaxing and socialising well. The common shared purpose amongst those studying medicine makes for a closeness which is one of the best things about life as a medical student.

The pre-registration house officer year and beyond

Applying for house officer posts

Most medical schools operate some sort of matching scheme in the final (or penultimate year). A house officer job-matching scheme does what it suggests – it matches prospective house officers to house officer posts. Some schemes are open to medics from any UK medical school, and some are only open to the university's own students. Some only cover the posts in the university teaching hospitals, and some cover all the hospitals in the region. Normally, the school which sends students to a hospital for clinical experience will supply the same hospital with its new house officers, but some schemes include posts that are many miles away. If you are clear that you want to work in a particular part of the country, it might be worthwhile finding out about the matching scheme. But remember that by the time you graduate the scheme might have changed.

The advantage of matching schemes is that some of the work needed to find a job is done for you and you will only be placed in university approved jobs. The downside is that some schemes give you little notice of where your first house job will be, or leave you feeling alienated from the process. Some medical schools produce too few graduates to fill all the regional posts and some produce too many, but for the foreseeable future medics have good prospects of getting work. If you cannot get a house job in the particular town or city you would like to work in, do not worry. During the training years you can apply for jobs elsewhere in the country (and abroad). Hospitals in Australasia, for example, recruit UK doctors for short term posts.

Registration

Graduating or qualifying from medical school with a **MBChB** or **MBBS** (or whatever) does not, in itself, allow you to practise medicine. First you must register with the GMC. Initially, registration with the Council is only provisional, but you can call yourself Doctor. To register fully you must complete two 6-month posts as a pre-registration house officer in surgery and medicine. Some regions offer house officer posts with 4 months each in medicine, surgery, general practice and other hospital specialties. House officer posts must be approved by the GMC for your experience to count towards full registration. If you complete these posts satisfactorily, you can apply for full GMC registration. Free hospital accommodation is provided for your job because the GMC believes that the right type of experience is only gained if you are resident, so don't worry if your jobs are in parts of the country you didn't choose. There will be accommodation provided.

Life as the house dog

The year as a house surgeon and physician is often the toughest in a medical career. There is much to do and learn and, sometimes, providing a service to patients and your employer is at the cost of your continuing education. You are well and truly at the bottom of the medical hierarchy, and demands from your patients, your colleagues and your bosses can be overpowering. Hours of work are long, (50,60+ per week) despite the European Working Time directive. Working intensively at night or weekends (on call) can be exhausting. As a house officer you will be responsible for taking histories from new patients, organising tests, following up consultants' instructions, helping at out-patient clinics and with theatre sessions. However, there are controls and ways of reducing the strains upon you. There will probably be times when you are fed up and may want to quit medicine. Some do, but the vast majority stay on. You will become more confident, more able to cope, and the work will eventually become more interesting (and challenging).

Beyond the house officer year

After the house officer year your career can begin to follow the path you want it to. For most junior doctors, this is initially in senior house officer posts through general professional or basic specialist training and, later, in specialist or GP registrar posts. If you have a strong idea what specialty you want to practise in, or you know you want to become a GP, then you can begin to take the appropriate path through the *training grades*. Don't worry if you do not know which branch of medicine you want to be in now, or even, for that matter, during the first few years after graduation. Many SHOs do not decide on their chosen career until well into their postgraduate training.

The two main areas of practice are general practice and hospital (specialty) medicine:

General practice

General practice is changing significantly but, currently, the majority of GPs are called principals. This means they are self-employed doctors contracted to work for a health authority. They usually work in groups which are small business partnerships. The most common route to becoming a principal is to do three years training as a GP registrar. This is divided into two years of hospital posts (in specialties such as general medicine, general surgery, A&E, obstetrics, geriatrics, or psychiatry) and one year working as a "trainee" in general practice. Most doctors training to enter general practice follow vocational training schemes in which the particular posts they will rotate through are pre-planned from the outset. By the time the latest entrants to medical school graduate, it is anticipated that a greater percentage of GPs will be employees rather than independent contractors.

Hospital medicine

Most doctors wanting to work in hospital aim to become consultants. To reach this level junior doctors normally rotate through two or three years of SHO jobs in medical or surgical specialities. After this and once their choice of specialty is clear, they spend between four and five years studying in registrar posts. There are specialist registrar "rotations" which allow a doctor to pre-arrange three or four years of training in different hospital posts. When this training is completed satisfactorily, a Certificate of Completion of Specialist Training (CCST) is issued and the doctor can apply for consultant posts.

Continuing medical education

Doctors must continue to study after they graduate and they are expected to keep their skills and knowledge up to date. This is a requirement from the GMC. The Council is introducing a system of formal reassessment for all doctors on its register – revalidation. Many skills and much knowledge will be acquired "on the job", but most career paths require some formal qualifications and exams will have to be passed. The Royal Colleges are responsible for medical education and for many specialties you will need to pass membership exams to get on in your career. In other specialties diplomas and Royal College membership exams are encouraged to supplement the minimum standards required. It was partly to encourage a positive attitude towards life-long learning that the GMC introduced changes to the undergraduate curriculum which foster learning skills and self-motivation.

Other career paths

General practice and hospital posts provide the greatest number of jobs for doctors in the health service, but there are many other career paths. Many doctors work in public health medicine, as medical academics, researchers for pharmaceutical companies, for the Armed Forces, and in private medicine. A great strength of practising as a doctor is the range of experience you can find in work. Flexible training is becoming more common and part-time posts are numerous. Many doctors have more than one string to their bow, and it is not uncommon, for example, for a doctor to mix private work or part-time work with their main NHS job. Putting together a portfolio career is possible as a doctor. A consultant might add some medical journalism and legal work in courts as an expert witness to their weekly duties as a hospital specialist; a director of public health might do voluntary medical work with a charity; or a GP might work part time with a local rugby club.

The following chart **Medical career structure** is taken from *Medical careers: a general guide*, published by the BMA (see *Further information* for details), and it shows some of the main career paths for doctors in the UK.

Medical career structure

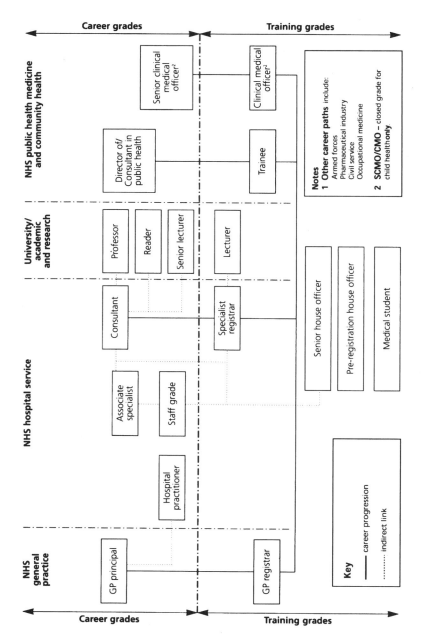

Medical career structure in *Medical careers: a general guide.*

The money question

It has always been expensive to study medicine, and with the recent government reforms it is now more expensive than ever. Medicine is a four year course at least and can be as long as six years, so you will have to sustain yourself, unpaid, for that period. The first two years are relatively easy, as a great proportion of your year will be holidays. For many, this allows living at home for half the year and saving some costs; also you will have plenty of time to earn cash in the holidays, if you want or need to. It gets more difficult in your clinical years (when you spend more time in hospital); a total annual holiday of six week's holiday is considered good! During this time you'll have to pay for rent and food for the whole year, and it becomes very difficult to work for cash having only six weeks off. Some students get part-time jobs during term time, although it is not always easy to find time to fit this in.

There are many kinds of expenses involved in studying medicine and debt is likely to stare you in the face a lot earlier than you may anticipate. Studying medicine is different from almost any other degree course and there are several additional expenses: for example, there will be many (expensive) books to buy – you could spend at least £150 a year – and medical equipment, such as stethoscopes, can cost between £50 and £60. You will need some smart gear once you're in hospitals regularly. This is not just to impress the doctors and nurses but to take on the guise of a member of the medical profession so that you will gain patient trust and respect.

The obvious question is: "How will I pay for all this?" The first port of call is your parents, guardians or family who may be able to give you something towards the cost of studying medicine. Problem solved if they are well off and generous, but if not (which applies to most of us) then there are government loans, bank loans, and overdrafts (further details below).

Some surveys suggest that medics graduate with about £12 000 of debt. A recent BMA report (*Annual Survey of medical students' finances 1999/2000*) found that the average total debt amongst final year students was over £9000. More than 21% of final-year medical students had debts in excess of £15 000. Although this may sound very depressing, please don't be put off studying medicine because of money. Yes, you are very likely to be in substantially more debt upon graduation than someone who takes a three-year degree course, but this is balanced by excellent future career prospects and good job security. Medical students come from all sectors of society, so if you weren't born to wealthy or generous parents, it's not a problem – you won't be alone in being in debt, and it won't be forever.

There are currently more jobs than there are doctors in the UK, and this trend looks set to continue for some time, so unemployment after graduation is not really an issue. Most medical graduates pay off their debt within five years of graduation, which helps to explain why bank managers tend to be very nice to medics.

Funding for the course

Tuition fees

Since October 1998, students have been required to contribute towards the cost of their education. For 2001/2002 the maximum home students will have to pay is £1075 per year. If your family income is below a certain level (approximately £20 000 pa) you will not be expected to pay tuition fees at all. The full amount will only be payable if your parents' residual income is in excess of £29 784. Tuition fees make up a proportion of the cost of your tuition, the rest of which is made up by your LEA in the form of mandatory and discretionary awards.

The BMA's Medical Students Committee persuaded the government that special consideration needed to be given to medical students because of the length and expense of the course and the Department of Health agreed to pay tuition fees for medical students from year five onwards. This will also apply to students doing pre-medical or intercalated years.

Living costs

Money for accommodation, food, transport, books, and beer will come from parental contributions, maintenance loans and (invariably) from banks. The amount of maintenance loan you will be entitled to will depend on where you study and what year you are in. These are administered by the Student Loans Company. Twenty-five per cent of the loan is means-tested and will largely depend upon your parental income. The maximum loan available in 2000/2001 for students outside London is £3815 and for those in London was £4700, with lesser amounts available to students living at home. Currently the amount that students are entitled to borrow in the final year of study drops by approximately £500 as the loan is not supposed to cover the summer holiday in that year. This hits medics very hard as towards the end of the course, holidays (an opportunity to make money) are much shorter and the final year of study can be up to 50 weeks long.

As a slight concession, in response to campaigns by the BMA's Medical Students Committee, the Department of Health has agreed to provide means-tested non-repayable bursaries for medical students from year five onwards which students will be able to apply for in addition to student loans. Students taking pre-medical and/or intercalated years will also be able to apply for this from year five onwards.

Student loan repayments will be paid in installments after graduation when your income is over £10 000 per year. For medics, repayments will begin during your first house office job which will generally be a few months after finals (normally starting in August).

Travelling expenses

Most of the teaching on the medical course takes place on clinical attachments in hospitals and GP surgeries. These can be quite a distance from your main medical school base and travelling expenses can be considerable. It is expected that most students will fund travel expenses out of maintenance loans although some of these expenses may be claimed back from your LEA. The rules currently state that you can claim back travelling expenses incurred in attending clinical placements although the first £250 must be borne by you.

Graduate students

Graduates will find that the arrangements for funding have changed quite dramatically for the worst since they were last at uni!

Tuition fees

Fees for graduate students or self-funding students on standard courses will vary from institution to institution (see later). Some institutions charge the standard £1050 per year whilst other charge more for the pre-clinical stage of the course and more again for the clinical stage of the course, so it is important to bear this in mind before applying. Graduates who have received support from public funds for the first degree are not entitled to receive any mandatory or discretionary funding from their LEA and therefore, would be liable to pay the full cost of tuition throughout the course. The MSC has been calling upon medical schools to limit the amount of fees payable by graduates to the standard £1050 but there is no guarantee of success.

In response to campaigns by the Medical Students Committee, the government has introduced concessions for graduate medical students on the four year accelerated degrees being held at Cambridge, St George's and Leicester/Warwick. Tuition fees will be paid by the Department of Health in years two, three and four of the course and therefore fees will be payable by the students in year one only. The MSC is trying to persuade government to extend this scheme to all graduate entrants to medical course.

Living costs

Graduate medical students are entitled to apply for loans from the Student Loans Company for help with their living costs. The maximum loan available in 2000/2001 for students outside London is £3725 and for those in London it is £4590 – 25% of the loan is means-tested and will largely depend upon your personal/spousal income. These figures are revised annually.

Graduates on accelerated courses can apply for funding to the NHS Bursary scheme in years two, three and four of the course. Graduates on standard courses will be able to apply from year five onwards.

Scottish students

Arrangements for Scottish students studying at one of the Scottish medical schools are slightly different.

Tuition fees

Following a decision by the Scottish Parliament to review student finance in Scotland, Scottish domiciled or other EU students studying at Scottish universities will not have to make a contribution to tuition fees.

The Scottish Parliament is considering legislation to set up a Graduate endowment scheme. Graduates would be expected to contribute a sum of around £2000 at some time after they have left university. The funds raised would be used to support future students. Repayment of the endowment begins after you start earning more than £10 000 per year (i.e. in your house job). The "St Andrews anomaly" where the pre-clinicals go on to do clinical studies elsewhere (usually Manchester) is yet to be settled.

Living costs

The Scottish Executive has introduced non-repayable maintenance grants of up to £2000 per year for students from families on low incomes. Access to maintenance loans from the Student Loans Company is also available.

Boosting your funds

Your friendly high street bank

In addition to the maintenance loan, a bank overdraft is likely to be required. Surviving at medical school makes this an almost essential part of your finances. Most banks and building societies offer students special terms on bank accounts. These normally include interest free overdrafts. Keeping your bank manager happy by not exceeding the agreed overdraft limit is good practice and also helps you avoid penalty charges and punishing interest rates. If you want to extend your overdraft, go and discuss it with the manager face to face. The bank wants your custom because you will have a good job at the end of your university career and they are experienced at helping students out with money problems. Banks are more likely to be generous and sympathetic with students who keep them informed than those who constantly surprise them.

If you need more cash than an overdraft gives you, then you will probably need a loan. Banks are more than willing to accept begging letters and IOUs from medics, and many have specially tailored loans of up to £20 000 for medical students. They often charge competitive interest rates. Remember that loans have to be paid back and interest will mount up. Make sure you fully understand the terms of the loan and shop around for the best deal. Don't just go to the bank you have an account with – it won't necessarily offer you the best deal.

Charities

There are literally hundreds of educational trust funds and charities in the UK. Many of these support medical students. They tend to be open to mature and graduate students rather than school leavers, but it may be worthwhile trying to find some funding from these sources. General directories of charitable trusts are available in the reference section of most public libraries, and some are listed in the *Further information* section of this book. Spending time searching through the lists and applying for grants may be to your advantage. Many small trusts have bizarre criteria for offering awards, and you may be surprised to find that by meeting the unusual requirements you can get help towards your expenses.

Access funds

Universities receive money from the government to help students in the poorest financial shape. Applications for the money are processed locally, and policies on how these are distributed vary widely from school to school. It is important to be aware that this money is available.

Work

For the majority of medical undergraduates, working during vacation time in the early part of the course is a necessity. As the course progresses, however, the holidays get shorter as term time extends and periods of elective study intervene and it then becomes more difficult to find employment for these shorter periods. You might consider taking a part-time job during term time. The medical course is undoubtedly challenging and demands a lot of your time in studying no matter how gifted you are. Because of this some medical schools discourage students from working during term. They cannot actually prevent you from doing so, but be warned they may take a dim view. Check out the school's attitude with the medics on open days. Do not let a job get in the way of studies.

A small number of medical students sign up to one of the armed forces (Air Force, Army or Navy) medical cadet schemes. A "salary" is paid to cadets for two to three years. In return for this support during undergraduate training cadets serve as an officer with, for example, the Royal Army Medical Corps, for a minimum period of duty (normally six years after full qualification). The income cadets receive is very generous compared to other students' incomes but the quid pro quo is the six-year short service commission. You will continue to practice as a doctor but the Ministry of Defence will require you to support military initiatives anywhere in the world. Working as a doctor in the Armed Forces can be very rewarding and challenging. It is the advice of the authors of this guide that students who embark on medical cadetships should be committed to a career in the services post graduation and not simply addressing the funding of their course. The forces recruit during the early years of the medical degree course and offer familiarisation visits for interested students. Contact details for each service are given in the *Further information* section at the end of the book.

Elective funding

Students who organise themselves well in advance can often get enough funding to pay for some (if not all) of the cost of their elective. You should have a wonderful time wherever you go, but it is so much nicer if you know you haven't paid for it all yourself. Depending on where you want to go and what you will be studying, there are numerous grants, research awards, sponsorships and bursaries available. Some will be open for all UK students to apply for and other funds will be distributed locally. Most awards and grants are given in exchange for some sort of project report or research work.

The final balance ...

Irrespective of your personal circumstances, studying medicine is undertaking a serious financial commitment. In common with many other students you will have to face up to some debt and financial worries. By accepting this reality and planning before you start how your tuition fees, parents' contribution, bank overdraft, student loan, and bank loans will fit together over the years, will help you to come to terms with it better. Make sure your acquaintance with debt is on your own terms.

Do not avoid dealing with tough money questions and do not adopt a head-in-the-sand approach to your finances. If you anticipate difficulties during the course, take advice from the Students Union welfare services, the university, and your bank. Don't leave it too late to take action – there are very few miracle workers and the people who are there to help are more likely to be helpful if they are given time.

This talk of poverty and debt is depressing, but remember these two things:

- Debt is now a fact of life for students, and the vast majority survive and free themselves from its tyranny.
- Medical students are better placed than most to pay off their debts at the end of the day, with excellent employment prospects and job security.

Applying to medical schools

Expansion of places

For the first time in many, many years the actual number of institutions at which you can study medicine is increasing. In 1999 the government announced an increase of 1000 places at medical schools. To accommodate this planned rise in the number of medics some schools have been allowed to increase their intake and three new centres of medical education have been approved. The new centres are at Durham, Keele and Warwick. They represent joint ventures with existing schools at Newcastle, Manchester and Leicester respectively. We have put some information about the courses at these centres alongside the information about the existing course at the partner institute. The majority of the new places have been added to the normal medical degree courses and those at Durham and Keele will involve periods of study at the new centre and also at the established centre. The new courses at Leicester/Warwick and St George's are specifically for graduate entrants and the first students began their course in September 2000.

New medical schools at the University of East Anglia, Exeter and Plymouth Universities, and King's College London (with the University of Kent), are opening with the first intake of students on the new courses happening in 2002. The new Welsh Assembly is considering how medical student numbers might be increased in Wales. Ideas include a school at Swansea or at Bangor.

Entry requirements

Most medical schools require students to get A or B grades (mainly As) in at least three A level subjects (discounting General Studies) or five Scottish Highers. Many schools also require the Scottish Certificate of Sixth Year Studies from applicants educated in Scotland. The entry demands have gone up as the competition for places has increased and the average requirement is now AAB (AAABB). Chemistry is usually a compulsory requirement because the principles of chemistry are the key to understanding medical biochemistry and it would be difficult to teach to the required standard during the course. Surprisingly, many schools do not insist on Biology, although many medics have it as one of their A levels. In most schools, medical teaching covers elementary biology and there may be supplementary classes for non-biologists during the first year if there is a need.

Traditionally, the other subjects studied at A level are Sciences or Mathematics, but many medical schools now acknowledge that students who pursue other subjects at school are not disadvantaged when they begin studying medicine. Some schools accept applications from students taking Chemistry, another science subject and an Arts A level. The key is to check closely with each school before you make your final choices.

In addition to academic qualifications, you will also have to fulfil certain health-related entry requirements. Individual schools have different requirements which they will inform you about if your application is successful, but in general you will need immunity against rubella and TB if you do not already have it. You will also need to prove your hepatitis B status before admission and, either before or immediately after admission, will be required to undertake immunisation. All health workers are required to have their hepatitis B status regularly tested as the disease is highly transmissible by blood and has potentially serious consequences. Hepatitis B carriers are excluded from performing blood-exposure-prone procedures and, in the unlikely event that a medical school applicant tests 'e'-antigen-positive, they will almost certainly be refused admission to the course.

The UCAS form – what they're looking for

Medical schools only accept applications made through the Universities and Colleges Admissions Service (UCAS). Read through the UCAS Handbook and follow the advice closely. Read the UCAS form and make several copies of it for practice entries. Your careers tutor at school or college will be able to help you fill in the form, but remember to make it accurate and legible. The most important part of the form is the personal statement. This is your chance to sell yourself to the admissions tutors and what you write will go a long way to deciding how many medical schools offer you an interview or a place. The comments below apply equally to electronic and paper applications.

You can expect – not surprisingly – that the medical school will want to know why you want to study medicine, and, as there is so much competition, you must seize this opportunity to demonstrate your commitment to joining the profession. For example, you may want to try to describe what drives you to pursue a career in medicine as opposed to other healthcare professions. However, don't take too much space to do this, as it will be at the expense of other important information. The challenge is to do this effectively with supporting evidence e.g. the hospital portering job, the auxiliary nursing you do at weekends and on Wednesday afternoons, captaining the school football team or designing the set for the school play. These examples will prove to them that you are a good candidate and that you are well rounded in your interests. It will be clear in the information supplied by your school or college whether you have got the potential to get the grades, so the personal statement must show you as a potential asset to the medical school and, later, the medical profession. They will be looking for signs of good interpersonal skills, evidence of a social life, details of your interests and hobbies, and any notable achievements. You may want to mention sports achievements, academic prizes, organisational or supervisory positions of responsibility, voluntary work, part time work, musical or travel interests, projects you have particularly enjoyed or unusual hobbies. If you are deferring entry for a year you should explain how you are going to use your time. There is no need to explain your choice of A levels unless you have something important to say about them. Allow yourself time to write as many drafts as you need, check everything ten times and then get someone else to. If you get called for an interview the panel will question you on the contents of this section so don't lie or exaggerate your interests or achievements. Remember, you may be asked to talk about any of the things you mention, so be truthful – it will probably show very quickly if you have embellished too much! (it is sod's law that if you say you collect Pokemon someone on the interview panel will want to know all about catching 'em all!).

Work experience is essential. Try to arrange work shadowing a local doctor, or in a hospital or nursing home. This can be difficult to arrange but keep trying. Auxiliary nursing or volunteer work will demonstrate commitment and enthusiasm; it will also give you some valuable experience to draw on in interviews and during the course.

Admissions staff read through hundreds of UCAS forms and if yours stands out then you will have a better chance of being called for interview. The admissions tutor will want to know that you are prepared for what a career in medicine entails and that you have realistic expectations, so by the time you post your application form you should have done your research and thinking.

You can use this book to help you decide which schools to apply to, but do not put an overt preference in the application. Another medical school may dismiss your application if they think that you will turn down their offer, and if you change your mind you will have limited your options. Also, think carefully about how your statement will appear to an admissions tutor reading it in his or her office. If you express a passionate interest in Scottish Folk dance a medical school tutor at Liverpool might think you would not enjoy being far away from the Highlands and not offer you an interview. Equally, an application to a London school might appear eminently sensible from a student wanting to see Fulham Football Club back in the top flight.

When to apply

Apply as early as possible, but do not rush your application form and remember the deadlines. Your form should be with UCAS before the 15 October 2001 deadline. The UCAS guide and website gives you all the details. You can submit your application electronically.

You may receive replies from medical schools virtually as soon as you apply or you may be kept waiting until the last week that offers can be made. Some schools may make a conditional offer on your application alone while others will conduct many rounds of interviews before they make offers or rejections. You may think you have been forgotten – this is very unlikely, but it does happen. If you are in doubt, and the deadline is approaching, contact the admissions office. You can arrange for UCAS to acknowledge receipt of your form, and you will be given an application number so you can check progress if you feel it is taking too long. Admissions offices will be very busy during this time, but a telephone call may put your mind at ease even if you they can't give you a decision on your application.

Gap years

Many sixth form students defer entry to university for 12 months. Gap years are looked on favourably by most colleges and universities. Most, however, expect you to use the time profitably by working and/or travelling. It is important that you check the medical school's attitude before you apply if you intend to defer entry. Time out between school and university is not just for those who have the dosh for a "round-the-world" air ticket. A well-planned gap year will give you time to think about how to get through university and let you assess what you want to get out of the next five or more years. Time spent well will boost your confidence and broaden your experience. This can have a very positive effect on your performance.

Student debt is increasing all the time. You could try to save some money and be in better financial shape for your eventual university career. A gap year may also be used to gain some more work experience in healthcare, although there is no need to overdo it, assuming that you gained some experience prior to applying to medical school.

NB: A minority of colleges at Oxford and Cambridge do not approve of gap years. It is best to check the attitude of the individual college(s) you are thinking of applying to.

The interview

If you are called to an interview, make sure you have done your homework. Interviewers will be looking at your form for inspiration on how to question and talk with you. They will probably be interested in what is special and unusual (but not weird) about you. Re-read your personal statement and anticipate the kinds of questions you might be asked. You should keep up to date with medical news stories and developments, as these may be the subject of some questioning.

Dress smartly and arrive in good time. If you are going to be shown around the medical school, remember that this is an opportunity to ask current students any questions you might have. Do not feel obliged to ask any questions in the interview, and do not ask questions which are already answered in the prospectus.

In some ways an interview is a way for the medical school to assess the potential it has recognised in your application form. It is not an academic test. Treat it as a chance to show that you are serious about your career choice, and that you will be a future asset to the medical profession.

Open days and further information

It is very important that you find out as much as possible about the medical schools that you are considering applying to. We have tried in this book to give you some of the available admission information and some views and opinions for you to consider. But it is only by visiting the place and reading the prospectus and any guides available from the medical school and the university that you will be able fully to assess the atmosphere and begin to see whether you will fit in. Open days will help you decide whether you would prefer a medical school that is part of a larger university, on a campus or spread across a town, in a big city or near the countryside, and where you'd like to live should you accept a place there. It will also allow you to talk to the medics who are already there. Starting university can be a daunting experience, but if you know what to expect then you will be much more at ease. If you can't afford the travel expense, get a group together and ask if your school or college will sponsor a minibus or take a coach load to an open day.

Most open days take place in the summer after the students have had their exams. It is better to go early before the students go on vacation rather than later. Open days over the winter tend to be more low-key affairs, but whenever you go, take time to have a good look around. Well-organised open days have a welcoming team to escort visitors from the station, organise events, talks, tours, displays and demonstrations. Dates of open days can be obtained from the medical school directly or via your careers tutor. Some medical schools run intensive open days during which you may have sample lectures. There are also one or two courses run commercially, giving an extensive insight into life as a medical student. These are sometimes expensive but can be a good way of deciding whether medicine is for you and you are for medicine. Your careers tutor might be able to help you find out about these events.

If you cannot attend an open day there are a number of people you could write to. The students' union can deal with enquiries and may have promotional material that it could send you. The medical faculty office should also be able to supply you with the name of the president of the medical society, the student group responsible for representing medics and organising sports and social events, so you can contact the students directly. BMA student representatives are always happy to answer questions and they may be contacted through the medical school or via the BMA Medical Students Committee (see *Further information*).

Mature/graduate entrants

More and more entrants to medical schools nowadays are mature students; medical schools view them as reliable and more likely to "stay the course". Many have done something else with their lives, often another degree, before taking the plunge into medicine. In some schools as many as 15% of students are older, and the staff are used to dealing with their different needs; in other schools older students are a rarity. The best way to find out if a school is "graduate-" or "mature-entrant" friendly is to go along and talk to staff and students. The expansion of medical student numbers has allowed the development of medical courses exclusively for graduate entrants. Leicester is running a four-year programme with Warwick University for biomedical science graduates; St George's has started an accelerated degree course for graduates called the Graduate Entry Programme (GEP), and Cambridge has about 25 places for a Graduate entry course starting in 2001.

Most self-funding students and many graduate entrants will incur higher levels of debt than their younger colleagues. However finances should not put you off applying to medical school. Far more important is your desire to study medicine and become a doctor. Competition for places is stiff, and many schools will not normally consider applicants over 30 years of age. Check before you apply.

Students with disabilities

The Disability Discrimination Act 1995 requires universities and medical schools to take into account the needs of disabled students. They must provide disability statements about facilities available for disabled students, which should include details such as access for disabled students, the specialist equipment and counselling available, admission arrangements, and complaints and appeals procedures for disabled students. The Act does not apply in Northern Ireland.

There are three main areas where disabilities may have an impact on medical work.

- The doctor's condition may limit/reduce/prevent him/her from performing the job effectively.

- The condition may be made worse by the job or make it unsafe for the doctor to do the job.

- The condition might make the tasks unsafe both for the doctor and fellow workers, or for the patients and the community.

There are many demanding aspects of medical work and any disability which may impede clinical capability needs to be considered carefully. It may be appropriate for students to have a skills assessment to ensure that they are fit to perform the tasks involved in becoming a doctor. This will focus on what the student can do, rather than what he or she cannot do. The medical school faculty and occupational health services may be able to offer skills assessment and advice.

Deans of medical schools should be able to offer further information and advice. Students may be eligible for financial help, such as the disabled students allowance.

Following the publication of a report from the BMA's Disabled Doctors Working Party called *Meeting the needs of doctors with disabilities*, the BMA has launched a service for disabled medical students and doctors who are BMA members. The service aims to provide information about aids, facilities, equipment and financial help. It will also put disabled medical students and doctors in touch with each other. Further information may be obtained from the Medical Education Department, BMA House, Tavistock Square, London WC1H 9JP.

Notes for overseas students

Applicants from outside the UK must apply via UCAS and should follow the instructions in the UCAS Handbook. You can get copies of the UCAS information from British Council offices or by writing to UCAS. Many schools and colleges will order supplies for you.

The British Council will have information about UK universities and medical schools. It will also be able to guide you on whether your qualifications are recognised in the UK. British Embassies or High Commissions and your own country's education authorities will be able to advise you on grants and scholarships. You should also make contact with your preferred medical schools directly. If you are not studying UK-examined A levels, then contact the admissions office at the medical school to check whether your subject choices and qualifications are acceptable. There are growing links between overseas medical schools and UK schools and you may be able to do some of your studies in the UK even if you do not get a full-time place on the course. If you are applying to medical schools in other countries you might want to enquire about this.

What if I don't get in?

The number of applicants to study medicine dropped more than 3% in 2000 to 9291. In spite of this and the increased number of places, medical schools in the UK are still vastly oversubscribed. There are often 10 applicants for each place. Only a small fraction of applicants will make it to interview, selected on the basis of their UCAS forms and references, even fewer will get a place. Oxford and Cambridge have a smaller number of applicants per place, which might mean that, although the academic requirements are high, you stand a slightly greater chance of at least being called to interview. However, not getting a place to read medicine is simply a reflection of the pressure on places and not a great indictment of your character and abilities.

Even if you maximise your chances of being selected for interview, you may still be unsuccessful in your application. You need to know what to do next. First, think long and hard! Do you still want to study medicine? Medical schools try to select people who will make good doctors and who have the right ability and motivations for studying medicine, but even so some medics choose to leave medical school mid-course and others fail exams. The interview panel has a responsibility to make the right decision for the medical school and you have a responsibility to yourself and your potential future patients to make sure you are making the correct choice. Examine your reasons for wanting to study medicine. If in doubt, or if you have felt pushed in the direction of medicine, it might be better to look at different courses or careers.

If you still want to study medicine, then start by asking yourself why you weren't successful in your application. Did you get an interview? If you did, your school might be able to get some feedback from the medical school. This is unlikely to be in depth, but might give you some useful information. Discuss the prospect of your chances with teachers. Reflecting on your disappointment at this stage may prove difficult but it is in your interests to be honest and realistic. Think about the possibility of following another course, whether in a related field – for example Physiology, Pharmacy, Physiotherapy, Biochemistry – or something totally unrelated. Most universities offer places on degree courses through "clearing". If your grades are good then many other courses will be open to you. Reapplication to read medicine is possible. Some schools will only consider a second application if you applied there first time round. If you do reapply, your A level results should be at least as good as the estimates that your school originally made. There are some schools which will consider resitting candidates. Save your own time and energies by asking your preferred schools if they would accept an application from you. This could prevent you from wasting future UCAS choices. It is only advisable to resit exams if you are sure about getting 'A' grades the second time around or if there were extenuating circumstances such as bereavement or serious illness in the months preceding your A levels first time around.

There are a growing number of places available for graduates to read medicine, which means that you could do a degree and see after graduation whether you still want to become a doctor. Graduates usually follow the full undergraduate medical course unless they can be exempted from part of the course because of the nature of their first degree (for example, Biochemistry or Dentistry). Graduates with a purely arts background at A level or degree could try to take a medical foundation year (pre-med year) before the medical course proper. This is not available at all institutions. Many schools do not normally consider applicants over 30 years of age. Graduate entry is, however, one of the ways into a career as a doctor. The BMA, and many other interested parties have recognised the desirability of graduate entry and it is sensible to consider this route as an option.

Pre-medical courses

Most medical degree courses last five years. However, some medical schools offer a six-year course starting with a pre-medical year. This year, which is intended as a foundation year in basic sciences, gives students with good non-science grades and some non-science graduates a way into the medicine degree course. Students who complete the year successfully can apply to join the medical degree course. Some schools allow automatic transfer to the first year of the five year course.

The exact nature of the pre-med year differs from school to school. In some schools it is taught within the medical faculty, while in others it is taught in other departments. Some schools offer exemptions from parts of the course if that subject has already been studied to a sufficient level, while others do not; and some schools offer a choice of subject, while others do not.

A list of schools that offer a pre-med course, and the respective entrance requirements, can be found in the table below. Some schools also specify that particular science subjects are needed at GCSE/Standard Grade level.

Medical school	No. of places	Entrance requirements (A level unless stated)	Contact for more details
Bristol	9	AAB	0117 928 7679
Cardiff	20 (medicine/dentistry)	AAB	029 2074 3949
Dundee	15 max	AAB AAAAB (Highers)	01382 344697
Edinburgh	10	AAB AAAAB (Highers)	0131 650 3187
GKT, London	45 (incl. pre-dental)	ABB	020 7848 6501
Manchester	20	AAB	0161 275 5025
Newcastle	10	AAB AAAAB (Highers)	0191 222 6771
Sheffield	20 max	ABB AAAAB (Highers)	0114 271 2142

Bristol

The pre-med year is spent studying the equivalent of A levels in Chemistry, Biology and Physics. Pre-medical students study alongside pre-dental students.

Cardiff

The pre-med year is modular. Students choose from a number of modules and the course is tailored to the individual's particular background. All modules are related to human medicine. A minimum of two sciences is required at GCSE.

Dundee

Dundee's pre-med students join with first-year BSc courses in Chemistry, Biology and Physics.

Edinburgh

The pre-med year consists of following courses from the first-year Biological Sciences course. The particular choice of courses depends on the individual student's qualifications.

GKT, London

Students study eight courses with pre-dental students covering Biology, Physics, Chemistry, etc. There are 45 places available. There is no quota for pre-medical places and places are filled on merit.

Manchester

The pre-med course has been redesigned so that students study in a problem-based style. Work focuses around problems or clinical cases. The course aims to prepare students for the new approach of the medical degree course. It gives students a basic grounding in all sciences, with most emphasis on Biology. Pre-medical and pre-dental students study together within the medical school.

Newcastle

Students study a combination of Chemistry, Biological Sciences and Medical Data Handling. GCSE passes in Maths, English, and at least one other Science subject are needed. Scottish students need to have standard grade Chemistry.

Sheffield

The pre-med year is spent studying Biology, Chemistry and Physics. GCSE Chemistry, Maths and English are required and Biology and Physics are preferred. The course is run at Barnsley College.

If the pre-med year is the only practical way into medical school for you, then your choice of medical school will be limited to those listed above. We suggest you make enquiries about the pre-med courses as soon as possible. You should find out about the funding situation from your awards agency and from the medical school.

Choosing the right medical school

By now you may be ready to draw up a shortlist of medical schools. There are many factors which might influence your choice of schools to apply to. Here are some final points to bear in mind before you start looking at the school profiles in our alternative prospectus.

The course

Although everyone needs to reach the same standard eventually, courses vary considerably. Don't, whatever you do, get bogged down in the minutiae of individual course descriptions in the prospectus. More often than not the courses on offer are subject to change, and many of us at medical school are on different courses from those that the prospectus had outlined. Here are a few things you might wish to consider.

Traditional teaching methods or problem-based learning (PBL)?

Traditional teaching relies heavily on lectures and practicals, whereas PBL relies on group work and individual study to a significant extent. This means fewer timetabled commitments, but you will have to sustain a lot of self-motivation. The more traditional courses will probably involve more basic sciences work and lab-based lessons. Anatomy has also seen many changes in recent years, with the dissection of cadavers by students being replaced, in part or full, with demonstration sections (or prosections) dissected by staff prior to class.

Exams and finals

Some schools have a greater amount of continuous assessment, which reduces the impact of finals at the end of the course. Decide whether you would prefer exams and assessments spread out or whether you would prefer to wait until everything fits into place at the last moment before sitting exams.

Special Study Modules (SSMs) and electives

Different schools will offer different amounts of time for you to study areas of special interest or to travel to work/study placements overseas. Some medical schools will allow SSMs in subjects such as history of medicine, medicine and art, and modern languages.

Holidays

Most courses last five years, but how the holiday periods within each year are spread will vary considerably. If this is important to you, find out how the individual schools arrange their vacations.

Intercalated Honours

UK medical schools take a variety of approaches to intercalated degrees. In some, the extra degree is open only to the academic high-flyers, some offer courses to almost any medical student while at others it is compulsory. If you anticipate being interested in some extra in-depth research leading to a qualification, or if you think you might like to follow an academic or teaching career, then think about this before you apply. Many medical schools allow students to study for the extra degree within other faculties of the university or at other universities.

Peripheral attachments

Most schools will send you away from the main university base for some modules. The distances involved can vary significantly. Are you the type who enjoys travelling and seeing different parts of the country or would you rather stay nearer your new home town and spend less on travel)?

Independent quality assessment of medical school courses

There are publicly available reports giving independent assessments of the quality of academic management and the standard of teaching and learning at universities in the UK. The Quality Assurance Agency (QAA) audits the performance of medical schools in England, Northern Ireland and Wales and its reports are available on its website. (http://www.qaa.ac.uk). Schools in Scotland are reported on by the Scottish Higher Education Funding Council and the most recent reports are also available on line (www.shefc.ac.uk).

The university

Although you will be applying to a medical degree course, a lot of the facilities and accommodation will be shared with a wider university community. Think about whether the medical school is on an out-of-town campus or based in a city centre or at a hospital. Do the medics mix with students from other faculties? The accommodation the university provides and where it is will have an important bearing on your experience of university, so think about what you want. You should also consider whether the university or medical school meets your needs in respect of sports, leisure and recreation.

The town or city

Wherever you end up, the chances are you'll be living there for at least five years (perhaps longer). It is vital that you choose a town or city that suits you. Think about whether you like the city and whether it will meet your requirements. Also think about how far it is away from your home. Long distances might be a disadvantage or an advantage: but remember, travel can be inconvenient, tiring and expensive. In later years, when holidays are in short supply, getting back for just a weekend may be difficult. Some cities are more expensive to live in than others but students can get favourable discounts and live reasonably cheaply somewhere in every city.

In most university towns crime is a fact of life and some of the entries mention this specifically. Irrespective of a place's reputation, you should always take care of your personal safety. You will learn quickly if there are any dangerous parts of a town or city centre which should be avoided when sorting out second year accommodation, so please don't worry too much about this.

NB: Wherever you go to study, please remember to register with a local doctor or the university health centre doctors.

The Insiders' Guide to Medical Schools

University of Aberdeen
Queen's University of Belfast
University of Birmingham
University of Bristol
University of Cambridge
University of Dundee
University of East Anglia
University of Edinburgh
Universities of Exeter and Plymouth (Peninsula Medical School)
University of Glasgow
University of Leeds
University of Leicester/Warwick
University of Liverpool
University of Manchester (Keele)
University of Newcastle (Durham)
University of Nottingham
University of Oxford
University of St Andrews
University of Sheffield
University of Southampton
University of Wales (Cardiff)

Medical Schools in London (University of London)
Guy's, King's and St Thomas' Hospitals Medical and Dental School
Imperial College School of Medicine
Royal Free and University College Hospitals School of Medicine
St George's Hospital Medical School
St George's Graduate Entry Programme

Please do not rely solely on the *Insiders' Guide* profiles in selecting your preferred medical schools. We have tried to be as accurate as possible with factual information and as up to date as we can, but if a particular piece of information is extremely important to your deliberations cross-reference or check it with the individual school's prospectus or admissions office. Remember:

- Read the medical school prospectus.

- Read the alternative prospectus (if available).

- Visit the medical school and the town/city.

- Visit the medical school website.

Note that the Average Cost of Living section is based upon 2001 prices. The cost of accommodation is sometimes given as within a range. Some of the more expensive rents in university halls may include catering costs. We recommend that you contact your LEA about the level of support you may be entitled. Also check with the medical school for the latest fee developments, as these are subject to change.

We have tried to lay out the information so that you can contrast the profiles easily, but if you have any suggestions to make about what we should or should not include in future editions please let us know at The Insiders' Guide, BMA Marketing Department, BMA House, Tavistock Square, London WC1H 9JP (e-mail to iurmston@bma.org.uk).

PLEASE CHECK IMPORTANT INFORMATION WITH THE MEDICAL SCHOOL.

885 students
Email: i.wells@admin.abdn.ac.uk
www: http://www.abdn.ac.uk

Aberdeen

The grey colour and cold temperature of the "Granite City" bear no relation to the warm and friendly atmosphere and busy social life that is Aberdeen. The age of the medical school is not reflected in the curriculum: a new integrated systems-based course which exploits technology to its full advantage; something that was commented on when Aberdeen was rated as excellent in a recent appraisal. Everything at the medical school/teaching hospital is on a single site (20–25 min walk from main campus), so you can go straight from lectures to the wards. Aberdeen medics tend to work hard, play hard and make the most out of being a large and distinct department within a university.

The course

The five years are split into four-phases. The phases are: fundamentals of medical sciences; principles of clinical medicine; specialist clinical practice; and professional practice. A core syllabus focussing on integrated systems for the whole class is counter balanced with special study modules for the individual. Students must complete each phase before passing on to the next. The first graduates from the new course qualified in summer 2000.

Teaching and assessment   Aberdeen was awarded top rating in the last Scottish Higher Education Funding Council Teaching Quality assessment. Problem-based teaching is partly replacing the traditional didactic approach and you will experience many different learning environments, such as general practice, specialist hospital wards, lecture theatres, and tutorial groups. Anatomy is taught by dissection and there is no compulsory use of animals in practicals. Computer Assisted Learning is integrated within each phase of medical training, supplementing the compulsory ward teaching and tutorials. Assessment is both continual and exam-based (written and clinical) with vivas for distinction and pass-fail candidates.

Placements outside the university   During the final two years you have the opportunity to study on attachment to hospitals in Inverness and Elgin. Moreover, GP attachments are now available throughout the North of Scotland, where free accommodation is provided.

Honours year   About one in five students do an intercalated degree (BSc) after year 3. You must have passed all your exams and not repeated a year to be considered. All intercalated students follow a core syllabus as part of their year.

Elective study/SSMs   All of the four phases of the course include SSMs, and in the final phase one SSM is non-medical. Students also have a 7-week elective period in their final phase, which can be spent abroad. This has a project component which contributes towards your final degree. It is not a holiday!

Course organisation   The course is well organised with distinct phases. Students must adopt a proactive approach, and self-motivation is an important requirement. There is a formal staff-student committee that meets regularly and a clinical staff/student committee that meets every five weeks to discuss the course. Different students are used each time.

Course details

Course length ●	5 years
Total number of medical undergraduates ●	885
Male/Female ratio ●	48:52

Admission procedure

Average A level requirements ●	ABB (Chemistry + Biology, Maths or Physics)
Average Scottish Higher requirements ●	AAAAB
Number of applicants (Sept 2000 entry) ●	1140
Proportion of applicants interviewed ●	All UK applicants + 20–30% of overseas applicants
Make-up of interview panel ●	Director of Studies for Admissions and 2 clinicians
Months interviews held ●	January–March
Number admitted (Sept 2000 entry) ●	190
Proposed entry size for 2001 ●	187
Proportion of overseas students ●	8%
Proportion of mature students ●	10%
Faculty's view of taking a gap year ●	Approved, provided you use the year well
Proportion taking Intercalated Hons ●	20–25%
Possibility of direct entrance to clinical phase ●	Very slim

Finances

Tuition fees per year ●	See *The Money Question* section
Fees for self-funding students ●	See *The Money Question* section
Fees for graduates ●	See *The Money Question* section
Fees for overseas students ●	£9000 p.a. (pre-clinical) and £16 920 p.a. (clinical)
Assistance for elective funding ●	Some funds and awards available
Assistance for travel to attachments ●	Minibus service
Access and hardship funds ●	Access bursaries and mature student bursaries

Average cost of living

Weekly rent ●	Halls £41–£86 Private £35–£60
Pint of lager ●	Union Bar £2 City Centre pub £2
Cinema ●	£3.50
Nightclub ●	£1–£10

PRHO year   A new matching scheme has been introduced Scotland wide in which the Postgraduate Deans ensure that there are enough jobs in Scotland for all Scottish graduates. Experience suggests that as the vast majority of the graduates want to stay in the Aberdeen area some will be disappointed.

The learning environment

Everything at the medical school is at the Forresterhill Hospital site so you can go straight from your lectures to your ward.

Library facilities   Good library facilities (open 8.45 a.m.-10 p.m. Monday to Thursday, 8.45 a.m.–8 p.m. Friday, 9 a.m.–5 p.m. Saturday and 2 p.m.-5 p.m. Sunday). Texts and journals are plentiful, as is access to Medline.

Computer facilities   There are many computers available with internet access, email systems, and good computer assisted learning packages for a variety of subjects. There is 24-hour access to computer labs at the university campus and at the medical school.

Clinical skills laboratory   A new clinical skills lab has just been sited in the hospital grounds equipped with all the up to date medical technology. It has been teaching senior medical students and junior doctors a range of clinical skills from venflons to defibrillation.

Teaching hospitals   Studying at one of the largest teaching hospitals in Europe allows Aberdeen medical students to experience a wide variety of specialties (including paediatric specialties at the Children's Hospital) on a single site. The learning environment is relaxed and friendly with the medical staff rewarding you with the help you need, so long as you put in the effort. Also, getting finals over with at the end of 4th year leaves time to earn up to £160 a week working as a student locum.

Student friendliness and support   There are regular staff–student liaison meetings, excellent relationships with lecturers, and the Dean is very approachable. There is a large support network should things go wrong: including academic tutors, individual advisors ("Regent Scheme"), trained counselling staff at the university, and the usual NUS welfare support.

Student life

The city centre is compact and lively with most pubs/clubs within 10 minutes walk of each other. Aberdeen is a prosperous town. The revenue brought in by the oil industry is apparent when looking at the excellent provision of shops, pubs, and other services. Because of this Aberdeen can be expensive to live in. As the medical school is isolated from other parts of the university, medics need to make a bit of an effort to meet with non-medic students, but the first year is normally spent in halls and this gives students an opportunity to network outside medicine. Most student social life tends to revolve around drinking!

Accommodation   University flats and halls accommodation are readily available for all years of study. The flats are generally nice but basic, and cost £41–£86 a week. There is a mix of catered and self-catering options. The vast majority of the university accommodation is centrally located, but some is a couple of miles out of town. Private accommodation is in high demand and can be expensive.

Entertainment and societies   The union runs many organised events and the Medical Society holds functions every two to three weeks and hosts an annual ball. University societies are numerous and healthy, covering a wide range of interests: sporting, dramatic, musical, outdoor, university armed forces units (army, navy and RAF), intellectual, malt whisky appreciation, etc. The medical school has a few societies of its own, and the annual medical revue is well supported and popular.

Sports facilities   MedSoc has its own rugby, football, cricket and hockey teams which compete against the other Scottish medical schools. The Aberdeen Medical Students Society (Med Soc) members can join an exclusive gym in town for a discounted fee of £80/year. The main university offers a wider range of sports. There are no specific medical school facilities, but the university offers inexpensive gym, pool, and tennis facilities to name a few.

City and surrounds   Just a short journey from the buzzing centre is the beach, with a new cinema, nightclub, and restaurant complex. In the other direction are the hills and the outdoors; excellent for walking, climbing, winter and water sports. The northerly location means the climate can be very cold, and, whilst there are road, rail, and air links, Aberdeen is a considerable distance from anywhere else.

The five BEST things about Aberdeen Medical School

- Friendly working environment and within a single site.
- Excellent student social life with civilised licensing laws (late opening).
- Easy access to the great outdoors (beach and mountains a very short distance away; skiing 45 minutes away).
- Long summer holidays when compared with many other medical schools.
- Good support network within the medical school and good staff/student relationship.

The five WORST things about Aberdeen Medical School

- No dedicated medics social centre on site.
- Cold in the winter.
- Travelling from Aberdeen often involves a long journey.
- Geographically isolated from the rest of the university, which means the majority of your student friends are medics. This is not helped by the different timings of exams and holidays.
- Our local football team!

Further information

Admissions: Deputy Director of Studies (Admissions) Medicine
University of Aberdeen
Academic & General Administration Section Registry
University Office
Regent Walk
ABERDEEN AB24 3FX
Deputy Directory of Studies Tel: 01224 272 035
Student Recruitment Services Tel: 01224 272 090 Fax: 01224 272 576

Belfast

Queen's University of Belfast provides a relaxed and informal integrated medical course. 90% of the students come from Ireland (both North and South), and a strong emphasis is placed on social life and enjoyment. The school also sits in a perfect position to access Belfast's nightlife, arguably the best in the UK. Queen's is the only medical school where it is not illegal to enjoy a good night's craic!!

The course

A traditional pre-clinical/clinical divide is less evident on the new course, and teaching combines a problem-based approach with more traditional lectures from the first year. Clinical skills are taught from year 1 in hospitals, general practice, and in a clinical skills centre. Each year is divided into two semesters and the trend is for year groups to be divided into smaller groups for teaching. In years 1 and 2 students learn the basic science of medicine with an integrated systems approach. The sociological and psychological aspects of medical practice are emphasised and Special Study Modules are taken. In year 3 the systems are taught again, but with an emphasis on mechanisms of disease. More time is spent in hospital attachments at this stage, and year 4 students spend all their time on the wards in hospital attachments or in general practice. The final year is a consolidation process with no new subjects.

Teaching and assessment   Teaching in years 1 and 2 consists of lectures, tutorials, lab practicals and meeting patients both on the wards and in general practice. There is a mixture of demonstration, dissection and prosection for teaching, and animal tissue is used in physiology. During years 1 and 2 only half a day a week is spent on the wards. In year 3 blocks of specialty-based integrated teaching is supplemented by pathology lab classes. Teaching is very much self directed, with the clinical aspects being taught on the wards. Years 4 and 5 are completely ward based. Computers and clinical skills are used for training and assessments throughout the course.

In the first 3 years examinations are at the end of each semester, whereas those in year 4 are at the end of each 8-week block. Procedure cards need to be completed as part of A & E medicine, anaesthetics, fractures and obstetrics, and gynaecology. Final examinations take place in two parts. The written examinations take place in September at the start of the final year and the clinical examinations are held at the end of the final year. During the final year the overseas elective, a clinical project, refresher clinical placements and a clinical apprenticeship are completed.

Placements outside the university   From year 3 onwards, hospitals and GP practices outside central Belfast are used. Hospital and GP accommodation is free and the furthest one might travel would be about 80 miles from Belfast.

Course details

Course length	● 5 years
Total number of medical undergraduates	● 877
Male/Female ratio	● 43:57 (starting year 1 in 2000)

Admission procedure

Average A level requirements	● AAA (A in Chemistry and another Science subject essential with Biology recommended)
Average Scottish Higher requirements	● Considered individually
Number of applicants (Sept 2000 entry)	● 521
Proportion of applicants interviewed	● 4% (QUB does not routinely interview pre A- level applicants)
Make up of interview panel	● 3 (Assistant head of School of Medicine, Director of Medicine, and lecturer)
Months interviews held	● February
Number admitted (Sept 2000 entry)	● 179
Proposed entry size for 2001	● 180
Proportion of overseas students	● 8%
Proportion of mature students	● 3%
Faculty's view of taking a gap year	● No problem
Proportion taking Intercalated Hons	● 5–10%
Possibility of direct entrance to clinical phase	● Transfers generally not accepted. There is a formal partnership with the International Medical College in Kuala Lumpur

Finances

Tuition fees per year	● £1050
Fees for self-funding students	● £1050 p.a.
Fees for graduates	● £1050
Fees for overseas students	● £9300 p.a. (pre-clinical) and £17 135 p.a. (clinical)
Assistance for elective funding	● Vacation Grant Scheme and faculty bequests are available
Assistance for travel to attachments	● Available through the Education and Library Boards for students entitled to a grant
Access and hardship funds	● Some university funds and bequests are available but amounts are small

Average cost of living

Weekly rent	● Halls £35–£55 Private £35–£45
Pint of lager	● Union Bar £1.60 City Centre pub £1.90
Cinema	● £2.50–£4
Nightclub	● £2–£10

Honours year   Between 5% and 10% of students take a BSc during their course, usually after year 2 or 3. Science degrees are available in Anatomy, Biochemistry, Physiology, Microbiology, Pharmacology and Medical Genetics. It is possible to study degree subjects that are not available at QUB by making arrangements with another institution. Approval for this, however, has to be sought from the dean. If there is competition for places, previous results in the respective subject will determine entry. Students from Northern Ireland may be eligible for LEA or bursary funding for the year.

Elective study/SSMs   During the summer vacation between years 3 and 4, students have the option to arrange elective pupilships for a period of 4–6 weeks at a hospital in the UK. In the final year students are encouraged to spend their elective period overseas. Students must also carry out a 6-week clinical project, either overseas or at Queen's, followed by the production of a project report of between 7000 and 10 000 words.

Course organisation   Course organisation can vary between specialties and ranges from excellent to ordinary. There is a degree of choice in some placements in year 4.

PRHO year   Graduates tend to stay in Northern Ireland for house jobs. Students from Queen's are guaranteed a house job in the Province. There is a surplus of about 15–20 jobs. Students apply to one hospital and are interviewed. If rejected from oversubscribed hospitals, students can then apply to an undersubscribed hospital for interview, and so on.

The learning environment

In years 1 and 2 most of the teaching takes place on campus in the Medical Biology Centre (MBC) and the Belfast City Hospital (BCH) beside it. These are about a 15–20 minute walk from the halls of residence. Other lectures and clinical work take place at the Royal Victoria Hospital (RVH), a 35–40 minute walk from the halls. However, a free bus runs from the BCH to the RVH every 15 minutes. Students from year 3 onwards receive teaching in the RVH and clinical attachments may be throughout the Province.

Library facilities   There are two medical libraries, the largest in the RVH, with a smaller library in the BCH. They both have on line catalogues, access to networked journals, and Medline and other databases. They close at 9.30 p.m. on weekdays and 12.30 p.m. on Saturdays. Study space is available at the Belfast City Hospital and at the Medical Biology Centre outside the library opening hours.

Computer facilities   There are eight computer centres with a total of 523 PCs, for use by all students. Their opening hours vary, but at least one centre is available between 8 a.m. and 12 midnight.

Clinical skills laboratory   A new clinical skills lab centre was opened in 1996. This is an essential resource for the new course.

Teaching hospitals   Ward group sizes in teaching hospitals tend to vary, but efforts are made to keep the numbers as small as possible to benefit both the patients and the students. The friendliness of the staff and their willingness to teach varies from ward to ward.

Student friendliness and support   Each medical student is allocated to a consultant who is known as their Faculty Tutor and is intended to help with any problems. The staff at the Faculty Office are friendly and approachable, as is the current Dean. The Students Union has a small counselling service. Rails, ramps and lifts are available in many areas for disabled access.

Student life

Although the capital of the Province, Belfast is more like a provincial city, small, lively, and not overwhelming. Everything you need as a student is within walking distance, and the centre of Belfast is only a mile away from the university and Medical School. There is a good range of pubs, cafes, clubs and cinemas (including a two-screen "arthouse" cinema). There are theatres, museums and galleries and most venues offer student discounts and concessions. Despite its reputation, Belfast in general, and the university area in particular, is a relatively safe place to live. Ninety per cent of students are from Northern Ireland with 1–2% from the rest of the UK and the rest from overseas. Medical social life focuses around the Belfast Medical Students Association (BMSA) which runs a wide-ranging programme of events. A key feature of Queen's is that the different year groups mix well.

Accommodation   There are places in university halls for every student who wants one. The rooms tend to be warm and comfortable with good food but thin walls. Catered rooms cost £46–£55 per week and self-catering rooms £35–£40 per week, inclusive of heat and light. They are about half a mile from the university. Biggart House is on the RVH site, which is very convenient for getting to ward rounds early but necessitates some transport (such as a taxi) to get to the main student area at night. For your isolation you pay £140 per month including electricity (but no meals). Private accommodation costs from £100 to £150 per month depending on the position and quality.

Entertainment and societies   The Belfast Medical Students Association (BMSA) is the oldest and largest student society in the university. Every year the BMSA runs a freshers' three-legged pub crawl, a mystery tour, a fancy dress party, the annual faculty ball, staff–student dinner, and regular discos which are attended by all years. The 4th year runs its own annual revue – tasteless but entertaining – and a medical charity called SWOT, which raises money by organising blood pressure clinics, street collections, a fashion show (with local TV celebrities) and pub quizzes. The Students Union has three bars and runs regular discos, balls and concerts. Like most universities, there is likely to be a society for whatever you want to do.

Sports facilities   There is a mens medics rugby team (the Spiros), which has an annual tour, a football team and a ski club which pays visits to the Belfast artificial slope. There are many sports clubs at Queen's, most of which compete in the Province's leagues. Near the university there are playing fields, tennis courts and a boat club. The Queen's Physical Education Centre has everything you need to keep fit. It is beside the university, well equipped, and costs 50p to get in if you are a student.

City and surrounds   Although you may have your hands full coping with what Belfast has to offer, it is easy to travel further afield. Dublin is just over 2 hours away by train and it is a must to visit the Giant's Causeway, the Mourne Mountains and the Fermanagh Lakes, all of which are within 1$\frac{1}{2}$ hours of Belfast.

The five BEST things about Queen's Medical School

- An updated curriculum in which students gain clinical experience beginning in year 1 with small group teaching.
- Queen's has an international reputation for trauma care, cardiology and ophthalmology.
- Belfast City is compact as a capital city but has everything you need.

- The social life – fortnightly events are organised by Belfast Medical Students Association (BMSA). Inter-year relations are good.

- Relaxed and informal atmosphere.

The five WORST things about Queen's Medical School

- The weather – there is no danger of students blowing their allowance on suntan lotion.

- The weekends tend to be quiet. Many students go home at the weekend, particularly in the 1st year.

- The siting of the main medical library means that at night students can only get to it by car.

- The ready availability of the "Ulster Fry" pushes your waistband.

- High number of students on some attachments.

Further information

Admissions: Admissions Officer
The Queen's University of Belfast
University Road
BELFAST
BT7 INN
Dean's Office Tel: 02890 245133 ext. 3477
Fax: 02890 330571
Admissions Office Tel: 02890 335081
Fax: 02890 247895

Birmingham

The medical school is situated at the west end of Birmingham University campus, just outside the heart of the city centre. Birmingham is a large provincial medical school that attracts a great diverse students from home and abroad. Its modern course is well established and produced its first graduates last year. The medical school has recently expanded and accepted 332 students in September 2000. Early clinical experience and the development of good doctoring skills is a key aspect of the course at Birmingham and admissions tutors look for well-rounded individuals not single-minded bookworms.

The school is lively in many respects, be it sport, drama, politics (medsoc!) or partying. From the first week as freshers, students at Birmingham can expect to work hard and play hard until their final year dinner held the week before graduation.

The course

Teaching during the first two years uses a systems-based approach. Regular patient contact in general practice begins within a few weeks of starting the course. Full time hospital teaching commences in the 3rd year in both medicine and surgery. Pathology and epidemiology are also taught during this year. Years 4 and 5 involve rotation through specialties such as paediatrics, oncology and orthopaedics in addition to senior medicine and surgery.

Teaching and assessment   Teaching in years 1 and 2 involves lectures and follow-up tutorials incorporating problem-based learning exercises. Modules are examined after Christmas and in the summer term by MCQs and short and long answer papers. Some in-course assessment is a feature of most modules. Students are expected to pass every module in order to proceed to the next year. Viva examinations may be held for borderline pass or honours candidates. There is no dissection at Birmingham, but we have excellent plastinated models to work with in a specially designed lab. Histology teaching is all done by video and accompanied by colour course booklets – there is no straining down microscopes for Birmingham medics! Hospital teaching combines bedside teaching, observation and participation in clinics and procedures. Clinical subjects are examined by MCQ and OSCE.

Placements outside the university   During years 1–4, groups of 4 students attend a local general practice once every fortnight. This offers a valuable early introduction to patient contact and clinical skills. A family attachment scheme is another community-based project that takes place in the second year. From the third year onwards, students attend hospital placements full-time for most of the year, with occasional teaching sessions in the medical school.

Intercalating opportunities   An increasing number of students at Birmingham are choosing to intercalate, typically after years 2 or 3. Options such as physiology, biochemistry, pharmacology or pathology involve a laboratory-based research project. Health sciences such as public health, law and ethics, behavioural science, or history of medicine are also popular.

Course details

Course length	● 5 years
Total number of medical undergraduates	● 1195
Male/Female ratio	● 44:55

Admission procedure

Average A level requirements	● AAB Chemistry (and one of Biology, Maths, or Physics)
Average Scottish Higher requirements	● AAAAB – must be Chemistry, Maths, Biology, Physics and English) (and 2 CSYS – any except General studies)
Number of applicants (Sept 2001 entry)	● 2097
Proportion of applicants interviewed	● c. 33%
Make up of interview panel	● Admissions Tutor, 3 staff, and clinical student observer
Months interviews held	● November–March
Number admitted (Sept 2001 entry)	● 336
Proposed entry size for 2002	● 330
Proportion of overseas students	● 10%
Proportion of mature students	● 3%
Faculty's view of taking a gap year	● No problem as long as there are plans to use the time constructively
Proportion taking Intercalated Hons	● 15–20%
Possibility of direct entrance to clinical phase	● No

Finances

Tuition fees per year	● £1050
Fees for self-funding students	● Please check with Birmingham
Fees for graduates	● Please check with Birmingham
Fees for overseas students	● £9300 p.a. (pre-clinical) and £17600 p.a. (clinical)
Assistance for elective funding	● Some competitive bursaries are available
Assistance for travel to attachments	● No
Access and hardship funds	● Some grants and bursaries are available

Average cost of living

Weekly rent	● Halls £54–£119 Private £45
Pint of lager	● Union Bar £1.60 City Centre pub £1.90
Cinema	● £2.50–£4
Nightclub	● £2–£10

Elective study/SSMs   Eight SSMs are completed during the course. There is a choice of many topics which, as the course progresses, have an increasingly clinical emphasis and become more self-directed. Electives are taken at end of the 4th year with an opportunity to travel anywhere in the world (some bursaries/grants are available but many students have to find some funding themselves). This normally lasts 2 months.

Course organisation   The course is now fully integrated. Lectures early in the course have a high degree of clinical relevance and topics are frequently revisited throughout the 5 years, therefore no single element of the course stands alone. Early clinical experience ensures that students definitely feel as though they are training to be doctors from day one. There is lots of scope for student input into how the course is managed through a staff–student consultative committee.

PRHO year   There is a matching scheme for PRHO jobs in the West Midlands. Most graduates choose and are able to remain in or near to Birmingham.

The learning environment

Situated in the suburb of Edgbaston, the university is just a couple of miles from the city centre. The medical school (which adjoins the Queen Elizabeth teaching hospital) is found at the west end of a refreshingly spacious and green campus. The medical school has benefited from the recent refurbishment and upgrading of lecture theatres, tutorial rooms, computer facilities and student common rooms.

Library facilities   The library is conveniently situated within the medical school and has an extensive range of medical textbooks and journals. It has plenty of quiet study areas and computer facilities with access to Medline, the internet and library catalogues. During term-time it is open from 9a.m.–9p.m. Monday–Thursday, until 7p.m. on Fridays and from 10a.m.–6p.m. at weekends.

Computer facilities   The ultra-modern computer cluster resembles a space station! There are currently just over 100 apple macs and 54 pcs in the main cluster. Every computer is online and allows full access to computer-assisted learning packages that supplement the course. Computer facilities are also available in general practices, teaching hospitals and in some of the DGHs that host student teaching.

Teaching hospitals   There are four large teaching hospitals in the city of Birmingham, as well as specialist hospitals and numerous DGHs. Medics at Birmingham will have very few long-term attachments outside the West Midlands and the majority of placements are within commuting distance of student accommodation.

Student friendliness and support   Pastoral care from a network of approachable student tutors is considered to be excellent at Birmingham. There is also an effective student run Curriculum and Welfare Committee that is respected by staff. The minder-mindee scheme that pairs freshers with a second year medic helps to orientate newcomers in their first weeks of university.

Student life

Not only is medicine the largest faculty in the University, but related courses such as medical science, physiotherapy and nursing are also based in and around the medical school. There is considerable social integration between all these students and between different year groups which has largely been attributed to the infamous Medbar. An enthusiastic medical society and final year dinner committee ensure there is always something happening and a good time is had by all. As the medical school is located on campus, medics can easily retain involvement in university activities and social events and therefore experience the best of both worlds.

Accommodation
Accepting a conditional offer from Birmingham guarantees a place in University hall/flats. All University accommodation is within 2-3 miles of the campus and most is within walking distance. The vale is a complex of several halls and flats which has the greatest overall capacity. The style of accommodation ranges from large traditional halls to flats with en-suite bathrooms. All halls have good security and excellent committees and social events.

There is plenty of private rented accommodation available at reasonable prices in Selly Oak - a mecca for students and just minutes away from campus. Selly Park, Harborne, and even Edgbaston, (which is, in parts, very posh) are also very popular.

Entertainment and societies
A very active medical society and final year dinner committee take care of the social side of medic life. This includes the renowned fresher's conference, pub crawls, wine tasting, curry quizzes, theatre trips, ski trip and a post-exam annual camping extravaganza to the Gower. Calendar events held in the medical school include the musical, review and final year fashion show. There is a huge annual medics ball as well as a summer ball and sports dinners. Many events are held in city centre venues which are easily accessible by public transport and fairly cheap for a taxi home. The Birmingham University Guild of Students (bugs) houses the usual complement of bars, clubs and pool tables as well as a society for every imaginable interest from rag committees to cocktail parties!

Sports facilities
The university has an excellent reputation for sport. The athletics union runs an impressive range of different sporting clubs! The medics also run large clubs for hockey, rugby and football, netball, cricket and basketball. Medics rugby, hockey and netball teams have all been national medical school champions in recent years. The clubs are friendly and well supported (especially in post-game celebrations) and cater for all ranges of ability, from absolute beginners to England players.

City and surrounds
Birmingham is indeed a cosmopolitan city. All the big name stores and designer shops can be found in the city centre as well as food to please every palate. Birmingham boasts a vibrant night-life ranging from the quintessential student night, jazz clubs to trendy bars and cafes that pop up on a weekly basis. There are plenty of theatres and the national indoor arena, NEC and Symphony Hall regularly play host to major international acts and are literally on our doorstep! The city and surrounding area are well served by public transport. There is in fact a train station just next to the medical school that connects to Birmingham New Street station and from there to just about anywhere. Birmingham International Airport is also accessible directly by train. More rural locations such as the Malverns, Stratford-upon-Avon and the Black Country are all easily reached.

The five BEST things about Birmingham Medical School

- Fully integrated new course with early clinical experience.
- Excellent relations between years and other degree students based in the med school.
- The (in-house!) Birmingham medical school med bar.
- End of rotation exams in clinical subjects instead of one-stop finals in the fifth year.
- Campus is great, compact and easily accessible from the medical school.

The five WORST things about Birmingham Medical School

- Having to do proper research during the elective (spoiling the holiday).

- The eternal traffic jam on the Bristol Road and M6.

- Med school administration....the wait for exam results, particularly in early years can be rather long.

- Some students feel that the amount of time allotted to general practice is more than necessary, although this module is currently under review.

- *Pulse*, the stomping venue of 70s night Carwash, once frequented by medics is....alas, no more.

Further information

Admissions: Admissions Tutor
Medical School
University of Birmingham
Edgbaston
Birmingham B15 2TT
Medicine admissions enquiries tel: 0121 414 6888
fax: 0121 414 7159
Prospectus requests: prospectus@bham.ac.uk

c. 850 students
Email: admissions@bristol.ac.uk
www: http://www.medici.bris.ac.uk

Bristol

Bristol is one of the old red brick universities but with a very modern course. As well as a close-knit medical school, there are numerous opportunities to enjoy a wide circle of friends. The city centre provides an excellent and reasonably compact environment in which to work and play. The university has a good reputation, which it justly deserves, producing high quality research and supporting generally good teaching.

The course

Bristol introduced an integrated curriculum in 1995. The integrated course consists of three phases. Phase I acts as an introductory period, lasting two terms, and provides a basic understanding of the human body and the mechanisms of health and disease. This is mainly taught in the School of Medical Sciences. Phase II lasts until the end of the 3rd year and consists of mixed clinical and theory-based systems-orientated teaching. Phase III includes teaching and clinical experience of specialty subjects (such as paediatrics, obstetrics and gynaecology). Also included are the elective period and senior clinical attachments in medicine and surgery. Clinical contact begins in general practices in the first year and the first hospital attachment is in the second year. Bristol also offers a pre-medical year to a small number of students each year, in which the teaching is with pre-dental students and provided by departments in the Faculty of Science.

Teaching and assessment   Pre-clinical teaching consists mainly of lectures and practicals, supplemented by small group tutorials and some self-directed learning. (No live animals are used in practicals, though occasionally some tissue, such as crab legs and guinea-pig ileum, is used in experiments.) Dissection room teaching is a part of the anatomy course, and is a very popular and rewarding element of medicine at Bristol. Clinical teaching is arranged around small groups which vary in size from two to around nine or ten (or more) and takes place in hospital and other locations, such as general practices and health centres. During phases II and III the whole year group is regularly brought together in Bristol for lectures and tutorial teaching. Regular assessments are made through the course. Many clinical attachments include projects or the preparation and delivery of a case presentation, whilst pre-clinical teaching carries associated tutorial and practical work. There are usually exams at the end of each year, though continuous assessment contributes to the final year mark. There are important professional exams at the end of the 3rd year and finals at the end of the 5th year.

Placements outside the university   Regional attachments occur from the 3rd year onward and are usually in district hospitals right across the south-west. Places like Truro and Exeter, the surfing paradise of Barnstaple, and towns to the north, such as Cheltenham and Gloucester are commonly used. General practice attachments are also spread across the south–west. Accommodation is provided wherever it is essential for students to be away from Bristol. However, although some help is given with travel expenses, travel to and from these attachments can be an extra expense (especially if you want to come back every weekend).

Bristol

Honours year   This is a popular option with about 25% of students opting to intercalate. The school positively encourages students to intercalate. The degree is normally taken after the 2nd year but it is possible to intercalate after the 3rd year. Students may choose a conventional science subject, such as Biochemistry or Pathology, though recently courses such as Ethics in Medicine have been introduced. The honours year gives students an opportunity to try some "real" science in the form of a potentially publishable research project as opposed to the rather spoon-fed medical course.

Course details

Course length	● 5 years
Total number of medical undergraduates	● c. 850
Male/Female ratio	● 50:50

Admission procedure

Average A level requirements	● AAB (must include Chemistry)
Average Scottish Higher requirements	● Please check with Bristol
Number of applicants (Sept 2000 entry)	● 1820
Proportion of applicants interviewed	● 20%
Make up of interview panel	● Academics
Months interviews held	● November–March
Number admitted (Sept 2000 entry)	● 149
Proposed entry size for 2001	● n/a
Proportion of overseas students	● 8%
Proportion of mature students	● 5%
Faculty's view of taking a gap year	● Positive if used well
Proportion taking Intercalated Hons	● 25%
Possibility of direct entrance to clinical phase	● No

Finances

Tuition fees per year	● £1050
Fees for self-funding students	● £1050
Fees for graduates	● £1050
Fees for overseas students	● £10 000 p.a. (pre-clinical) and £18 710 p.a. (clinical)
Assistance for elective funding	● No
Assistance for travel to attachments	● Some
Access and hardship funds	● Some grants and bursaries

Average cost of living

Weekly rent	● Halls £34–£90 Private £42–£65
Pint of lager	● Union Bar £1.50 City Centre pub £2.20
Cinema	● £3–£5
Nightclub	● Free–£8.00

Elective study/SSMs   SSMs are an important part of the new curriculum from the first year onwards, allowing students to pursue subjects of special interest. Elective time is currently during the 5th year. Arrangements regarding the elective may be subject to change so check with the university for further information.

Course organisation   Individual biomedical departments run their own courses but communication between departments is good and the separate elements of the course are integrated well. Some departments assign hospital placements, but many offer some sort of choice. Departments generally try to accommodate students with special requirements (for example parents with children).

PRHO year   There is a matching scheme run from Bristol that includes most of the jobs in the south-west. Almost all students enjoy their time at Bristol, and many stay on in Bristol during the holidays as there is plenty of temporary work to be found. A lot of graduates stay in the Bristol area after graduation.

The learning environment

The first two years are spent mainly around the university campus in central Bristol. When you begin clinical specialty attachments, you can be placed at one of the main Bristol hospitals or anywhere throughout the south-west – including as far away as the surfing towns in Cornwall.

Library facilities   The medical library is open until 9 p.m. on weekdays (5 p.m. or 6 p.m. during the long vacation) and on Saturday mornings. The main library has longer opening hours. Popular textbooks are available from the medical library on a short loan basis. Medline, Embase and other databases are on open access in libraries, and email and internet connection are also available there and in the halls of residence.

Computer facilities   Computers are available in the Medical School (including the library) and in the main library. There are a number of 24 hour open access rooms dotted around the university. Computer-assisted learning packages are available in the medical library. Other terminals support internet access, email, word processing, etc. Information technology is supposed to be an integral part of the new course, but at times teaching can be of poor quality and the quality of computing facilities is variable.

Clinical skills laboratory   This is situated in one of the main teaching hospitals in Bristol, the BRI. In the 2nd year adult life support is taught and students are examined and certified. The clinical skills lab is also used to teach venepuncture to 2nd year students. As students progress through the course, other clinical procedures, such as intubation, may be learnt here.

Teaching hospitals   Students are divided among the three big hospitals in Bristol. These are generally friendly, some more than others. Teaching groups can range in size from two to eight. Outside the Bristol hospitals groups tend to be smaller, allowing more time for individuals to learn.

Student friendliness and support   A personal tutor scheme operates and it normally works well. The variable quality of the scheme depends on the tutor (and tutees). However, most students find a member of staff with whom they get on well and from whom they can seek help. The Faculty tends to be supportive, provided they are informed of problems before they get out of hand. There is a staff–student liaison committee, but input does not often translate into immediate action. The university and the Students Union both have counselling services. Access for students with disabilities may be difficult because of the layout of the university (on a steep hill). The secretary of Galenicals (the medical students society) is also there to voice student opinions and views to the Medical School.

Student life

Bristol has a lot to offer both as a university and a city. The university is a research-orientated institution with a good reputation but also provides good teaching. The city is just brilliant fun. Mainstream attractions abound and there is plenty of "alternative" entertainment for those who want it. It is still a reasonably safe city (at least in the areas frequented by students) providing appropriate precautions are taken. It is certainly no worse than most other cities in this respect. If city life becomes too hectic, there are plenty of green spaces to escape to.

Accommodation   Most first years are accommodated in university halls of residence. These tend to be comfortable enough and provide an excellent opportunity to bond with other freshers (medics and non-medics) at the numerous organised events or in the hall bars. The main group of halls is located a 30–40 minute walk from the university precinct. It is possible to apply to stay in hall after the 1st year, but most people move into university flats/houses or into accommodation in the private sector. Weekly rents vary between £45 and £60 or more, but most students pay between £50 and £55. It is usual to pay rent over the summer and the scrum for houses starts quite early in the year. The accommodation office provides some help but a lot depends on individual initiative.

Entertainment and societies   Entertainment abounds in Bristol - sometimes there seems to be too much choice! A number of big acts play at the university and at other venues throughout the city. There is a huge range of societies to join at the Union. Halls and Galencials lay on a range of entertainment, organise a number of sports teams and represent students' views on a variety of committees. There are two revues for medics to take part in. The pre-clinical revue tends to be a rather drunken and disorganised affair, but the clinical one is a more organised and moderate event which runs for four nights in the Union theatre. Galenicals organises a lot of events for medics and has its own bar which students from all year groups use.

Sports facilities   The university has good outdoor facilities, a new indoor tennis centre and plans are well under way to develop a new indoor centre within the campus. Wednesday afternoons are usually free for sport and there are teams at all levels in most sports. There are a number of medics' teams (including the infamous Women's Football Team) organised through Galencials, which tend to be a bit less competitive than the university teams. They have a considerable social component (and alcohol consumption, too!).

City and surrounds   The city centre is reasonably compact and packed with things to attract all comers. The countryside (and attractions of the West Country and Wales) is not far away. Students tend to congregate in the areas just around the university, such as Clifton. However, there is a shift towards areas a little further away which offer cheaper rents. Clifton is the most affluent (and "posey") part of Bristol, offering pleasant cafes and bijou shops. Town and gown tension is rarely a problem. Shopping, theatre, museum and music lovers will all find something up their street. There are plenty of pubs, restaurants, clubs, cinemas (including three "arthouse" cinemas), plenty of parks and green spaces, and all the other things you would associate with a vibrant city like Bristol.

The five BEST things about Bristol Medical School

- Friendly and close-knit medical school.
- The generally high standard of teaching and the high quality of clinical experience, especially in peripheral hospitals.
- The city of Bristol itself – with its huge range of bars, restaurants and attractions.

- The opportunity to mix with plenty of non-medics and medics from other year groups.

- A modern, clinical course in which student feedback is valued.

The five WORST things about Bristol Medical School

- The rather conservative nature of the university in terms of atmosphere and politics.

- The financial costs (high rents; long distance attachments in clinical years; expensive bus fares).

- Walking up all those steep hills (Bristol is one big hill).

- Feedback on exams you have just taken can sometimes be a bit limited.

- Huge scramble for accommodation at a reasonable price.

Further information

Admissions: Undergraduate Admissions Office
University of Bristol
Senate House
Tyndall Avenue
Bristol
BS8 ITH
Admissions Office Tel: 0117 928 7679
Fax: 0117 925 1424

Bristol

Cambridge

Following a traditional format, the Cambridge course is a fast-track, intensive course which places much emphasis on understanding the principles behind biological science and its application to medical practice and research. What makes the Cambridge course stand out from most of the others is the supervision system at both the pre-clinical and clinical stages (see teaching and assessment below). The medics tend to be a social group, mixing well with each other and students on the other courses. Life is rarely dull and there is always plenty to do within the colleges, the university and the city.

Cambridge Graduate Course

Cambridge's innovative contribution to the expansion of medical student places has been to offer a four year MB/BChir course to graduate entrants. The first students will start their studies in 2001. The course is the result of a partnership between Cambridge University and the West Suffolk Hospital and local General Practices in Bury St Edmunds. Clinical and communications skills are taught from early on and the course is structured around vertical strands such as clinical skills. The course seeks to integrate the practice of medicine with the study of core medical sciences. Medical science will be studied in Cambridge and clinical training will be in and around Bury St Edmunds. Purpose-built residential and teaching accommodation is being built at the hospital.

Applications are welcomed from graduates with a first class or upper second class degree in any subject. All candidates have to sit the MVAT (Medicine & Veterinary Admissions Test). The course is only open to students who are classified as Home or EC. There are currently 20 places on the course.

For more details visit the website (**www.medschl.cam.ac.uk**)

Intercollegiate Admissions Office www.cam.ac.uk/CambUniv/undergrad

---

The course

The pre-clinical and clinical stages are very distinct and separate. The pre-clinical course is divided into two parts. In Part I, which lasts two years (40 weeks, really!) and during which all the 2nd MB exemptions are usually gained, the teaching covers the topics of anatomy, biochemistry, endocrinology, genetics, pathology, pharmacology, physiology, population sciences, psychology, neurobiology and reproductive biology. (Some of the practicals in Part I use freshly killed animal specimens.) Part II, the 3rd year, is essentially equivalent to the intercalated BSc elsewhere and leads to a BA (Hons). Students are technically allowed to study any subject they choose, though this needs to be "medically related" if they wish to do a short clinical course and stay on in Cambridge. During the pre-clinical course, students get very little exposure to hospitals and the course is based in the centre of town where the various science faculties are situated. However GP shadowing visits have now been introduced to the pre-clinical course. Also at the end of each term in year one the clinical school arrange for students to be presented with patients who have injury or pathology relevant to that terms anatomy/dissection.

The clinical stage, which is based at Addenbrooke's Hospital, is intensive, lasting only 27 months, and is divided into three phases, during which time attachments to all the major specialties are organised. Final MB examinations in Pathology and Obstetrics & Gynaecology are taken at the end of Phase II (after 18 months of the clinical course) and the remainder at the end of Phase III. Most of the work is ward-based and students are expected to be proactive. There are lecture blocks throughout the course but these are kept to a minimum. It should be remembered that there is non-automatic progression to the clinical school and only about half the Cambridge pre-clinical students stay on although last year all students who wanted to stay on were able to do so. The rest normally go to the London Schools or Oxford, but it is also possible to go to Edinburgh or other medical schools with compatible courses to undertake clinical studies.

The university now sets an admissions test for all applicants to all colleges. This test is sat at the student's own school. It consists of multiple choice questions (sections A and B) and two essays from either Maths, Biology, Chemistry or Physics and takes two hours in total. The test is designed to make you think and reason clearly about particular topics and is not a test of factual knowledge. It is set to require no knowledge beyond key stage 4 of the National Curriculum and should not stop anyone from coming here. Everyone that applies is still interviewed and for the next couple of years the examiners do not intend the test result to form a large part of the criteria upon which the offer a place is made.

Teaching and assessment   During the pre-clinical stage the teaching programme consists of lectures (with the occasional seminar) and practicals (which must be attended) organised by the medical sciences departments. These are supplemented by weekly small group tutorials (consisting of two or three students) known as supervisions, which are organised by the individual colleges. Formal assessment is in the form of end of year examinations. These are essay or theoretical experimental practical papers, but a few are actually practical papers. During the anatomy course there are occasional informal "sign up" or viva tests which do not contribute to the end of year grade but ensure that you are keeping up to date with the work. In Part II, a research project or dissertation may contribute to your classification.

The majority of teaching in the clinical stage is ward based. The medical firms for each attachment consist of two to six students and there is an assessment of progress at the end of most attachments. Formal assessment, vivas and written exams occur at the end of each phase. A doctor arranges weekly clinical supervisions to monitor/guide the student through the entire course. Some emphasis is based on computer-assisted methods of learning and students are expected to be reasonably computer literate by the end of the course.

Placements outside the university   There are regional attachments in up to a maximum of six out of the 11 Phase I and II placements. In Phase III, half of the time is spent at Addenbrooke's and half in a district general hospital. Accommodation at these placements is provided.

Course details

Course length	• 5 ½ years
Total number of medical undergraduates	• c. 767 pre-clinical, c. 387 clinical
Male/Female ratio	• 47:53 pre-clinical, 71:59 (1999 clinical entry)

Admission procedure

Average A level requirements	• AAA (in Sciences/Maths – some colleges ask for STEP papers)
Average Scottish Higher requirements	• Check with individual college admissions tutors
Number of applicants (Sept 2000 entry)	• Pre-clinical: 1189 Clinical: 139
Proportion of applicants interviewed	• Pre-clinical: 99% Clinical: all applicants choosing Cambridge as first choice, plus others at Dean's discretion
Make up of interview panel	• Pre-clinical: this varies from college to college from being very informal to having written tests; 2–4 interviews may be required Clinical: Three members of the clinical teaching staff; single 15-minute interview
Months interviews held	• Pre-clinical: December prior to A levels Clinical: January prior to final (3rd year) undergraduate exams
Number admitted (Sept 2001 entry)	• Pre-clinical 268 Clinical 130
Proportion of overseas students	• Pre-clinical: 18 Clinical: 18 (1999 entry)
Proportion of mature students	• Pre-clinical: 12 Clinical: 7
Faculty's view of taking a gap year	• Dependent on individual college
Proportion taking Intercalated BSc	• None; all students study for 3 pre-clinical years including a BA (Hons)
Possibility of direct entrance to clinical phase	• All students are interviewed again before entry to clinical school. About 10% of clinical school intake is from other UK medical schools

Finances

Tuition fees per year	• £1050 + c. £2900 college fees (paid for all non-graduate home students)
Fees for self-funding students	• Pre-clinical £1050 p.a. Clinical £2610 p.a.
Fees for graduates	• Please check with Cambridge
Fees for overseas students	• Pre-clinical £9042 p.a. Clinical: £16 734 p.a.
Assistance for elective funding	• There are a limited number of bursaries
Assistance for travel to attachments	• Only available to LEA-funded students
Access and hardship funds	• Dependent on individual college

Average cost of living

Weekly rent	• Halls £30–£50 Private £40–£60
Pint of lager	• Union £1.50 City Centre pub £2
Cinema	• £1.50–£3.80 (with student card)
Nightclub	• £1 (before 10.30 p.m. on student nights)–£5

Honours year   All students must complete the 3rd year (Part II), which leads to a BA (Hons) in the subject in which they have specialised.

Elective study   The elective study takes place after the Final MB exams at the end of Phase II. It is 7 weeks in duration, with 95% of students going abroad. Limited funding is available for electives from the clinical school, though students have to compete for these (value £80–£200, total £2000), and there may also be some assistance from your college (value dependent on the college).

Course organisation   On the whole, the course at the pre-clinical level is very well organised. The quality of clinical teaching is, like everywhere, dependent on the firm you are attached to for each placement – this tends to be usually very good. Students are generally well informed of where they should be and what they should be doing. However, there is no choice of placements for students – you go where you are told!

PRHO year   The majority of clinical students stay on for regional house jobs. There is a very comprehensive matching scheme and most students are found placements after qualification.

The learning environment

The pre-clinical lectures, seminars and practicals are all held in the science faculty away from the hospital and all within walking distance of the central colleges. The tutorials are usually held within your own college. Very few teaching sessions are held in the hospital during the pre-clinical stage. During the clinical stage, all the teaching is done at Addenbrooke's which is situated $2\frac{1}{2}$ miles from the city centre and can be easily reached by bus or cycle (20 minutes) if you are not able to get a lift with a friend.

Library facilities   You cannot go anywhere in Cambridge without being fairly close to a library; all the colleges, departments and faculties have them. There is also a central university library, central city library and a specialist medical library at the clinical school, so the chances of not being able to get hold of a particular book or paper is almost zero. All of the libraries are open during office hours and some have 24-hour access.

Computer facilities   As with the libraries, there are computing facilities everywhere; everyone is given an email account as well as college and university log-ins. Basically they are excellent. Most colleges have university network connections to some of the undergraduate rooms.

Student friendliness and support   Administration of the pre-clinical course is at college and university level, but all students are given a tutor (a non-medical fellow), who is responsible for their pastoral care, and a director of studies (medical fellow), who is concerned with ensuring they receive the appropriate academic help. The Clinical Dean is also friendly and helpful.

Student life

Cambridge life is a heady mix in terms of inhabitants and surroundings. The collegiate system means that in the pre-clinical years you get to meet students doing a wide variety of subjects and not just medics. Though the course does place a workload on you, there is time to do plenty of other things, especially sport and music which are well represented throughout the university. There is much more of a "medical school" feel to the clinical stage, with most students living nearer the hospital and away from their colleges. The small batch size means that by the end of the course everyone gets to know one another.

Accommodation

The quality and the cost vary with the college (and the wealth of the college), so choose wisely, especially if you are a clinical or overseas student. All of the colleges will provide accommodation in or close to college for the pre-clinical years, and most will provide accommodation for the clinical years. The standard at its worst is definitely bearable. At its best, you are unlikely to get better rooms anywhere else, and it is probably better than your own room at home! During the clinical stage you may have to rent accommodation from local landlords and this costs between £50 and £60 per week for a middle of the range house usually shared by three or four people.

Entertainment and societies

Entertainments are provided at a variety of levels, and may be society, college, clinical school or university based. If that is not enough, then there are many shows and concerts put on by non-university establishments within the town. If this is still not enough to satisfy your needs (which means you are probably not doing enough work!), you can head into the centre of London in about forty minutes. The University Medical Society is the fourth largest and works to make sure medics have a good time. Every year there is a Christmas dinner, and other activities such as bops, barbecues and pub-crawls are also organised. On top of this, there is a whole host of opportunities to be involved with in other societies, from drama and music to karate and gliding, so the chances are you can find something you will enjoy doing.

Sports facilities

Almost every sport is catered for at the university level. Facilities at college level vary, but at best include huge playing fields, a multigym and squash courts. Boat clubs, football, rugby and cricket tend to have the largest shares of the college budgets. Also, it does not matter how good you are, there is always an opportunity to take part in whatever you choose. During the pre-clinical stage, sport is college based and there is fierce inter-collegiate rivalry. The clinical school has a sports society (known as "the Sharks") and there is a sport and fitness centre situated on the hospital site to which all students are given free membership.

City and surrounds

With its undeniable beauty and rich history, Cambridge is an inspiring city to work and live in. Undergraduates during term time, graduates and tourists at all times and, of course, the local residents (affectionately known as "townies") provide an ever changing and colourful population superimposed on secluded college cloisters, colonies of student houses and a busy town centre. On a more practical note, all the usual student needs are provided for within a 15-minute cycle ride or less. Take your pick from the covered central market, essential supermarkets and a wide range of chain stores, to the excellent Arts Theatre, Corn Exchange and Guildhall, as well as a number of cinemas - college, arthouse and mainstream. The river soon meanders to open countryside in either direction and, finally, many routes lead out of Cambridge to London (and its attractions) as well as the rest of the country.

Cambridge is not without the dangers of violence and crime and, like most places, these problems are often associated with last orders on a Friday or Saturday night. However, there are no notorious districts and students' property insurance premiums confirm Cambridge as one of the safest places to live and study.

The five BEST things about Cambridge Medical School

- The collegiate system means that you get to meet students doing a wide variety of subjects, and predisposes you to a broader education.

- The supervision system ensures that you are able to get help with any academic difficulties, helps to make sure that you are able to keep up with the course and gives you substantially more individual tuition than most medical schools.

- The medical societies organise a wide variety of events on a regular basis and the medics are renowned for being a very sociable bunch – and drinking far too much!

- The breadth and quality of the extra-curricular activities available and the diversity of the interesting people you meet whilst in Cambridge makes it truly unique.

- The cost of living is relatively low, and the proximity of all the necessary amenities makes Cambridge an ideal place to spend life as a student.

The five WORST things about Cambridge Medical School

- Cambridge is a very competitive learning environment, especially just prior to exams, and some students can find this stressful.

- There is a lot of emphasis on teaching the medical sciences in great detail in the pre-clinical stage, and some students get frustrated by this.

- The course is intensive and it may be easy to fall behind. Though the pre-clinical terms are short (only 8 weeks of study), they can be very tiring, but this is made up for by longer holidays.

- The small size of the town can make life feel somewhat claustrophobic at times.

- The tourists – though they do admittedly generate a lot of income for the town and the colleges – tend to get under your skin and manage to appear almost anywhere and at any time (including occasionally in lectures!)

Further information

Admissions: Cambridge Inter-collegiate Admissions Office (CIAO),
Kellet Lodge
Tennis Court Road
Cambridge CB2 1QJ
Tel: 01223 333308
Fax: 01223 366383

Cambridge

Dundee

Dundee is a progressive, modern, friendly, forward-thinking medical school with an international reputation. The new curriculum was introduced in 1993. Dundee medics have a reputation for being friendly and down to earth. Intake is approximately 40% Scottish, 40% Irish, 10% English and 10% overseas. Dundee is extremely supportive of graduate/mature students and encourages applications from a wide variety of backgrounds. Over 16% of every year are graduate/mature students, and each year also has about seven entrants from the pre-med course.

The curriculum offers good staff–student participation and has achievable learning goals with a realistic workload. Clinical teaching begins in the second year. Many aspects of the course at Dundee have received plaudits from the Scottish Higher Education Funding Council. The biomedical research programme is world renowned. Ninewells Hospital, the largest purpose-built teaching hospital in Europe, is built on a green park campus on the banks of the River Tay.

The course

The class of 2000 was the first to graduate having followed the new curriculum and the course is well established. Teaching is structured around body systems. The first year (Phase 1) covers normal structure and function and is taught at the main campus. First year students also visit patients in the community and do a basic CPR course. During first year students are divided into groups for tutorials and practicals. Groups change in the second year for the Practising Medicine (clinical) programme, which helps you get to know more of your year. Phase II (second and third year) and III (fourth and fifth year) are based at Ninewells Hospital. The curriculum requires mastery (a pass grade of 75%) of relevant facts, clinical skills, and attitude. Special Study Modules are a key component, but are assessed using different criteria.

Teaching and assessment   The systems-based course promotes independent learning. Each block comes with a study guide, which includes core material and a summary of the clinical skills to be mastered each week, problem-based questions, tutorial questions and references. Phase I teaching is a mixture of lectures, dissection, labs, behavioural sciences and tutorials. There is no use of animals or animal tissues in practicals. Phase II includes clinical skills, ward teaching (approx. eight students to a ward group), small group work and primary care medicine. Phase III is primarily clinical and includes a house officer apprenticeship in the fifth year. This provides extensive training so that students will be competent and useful HOs, and often occurs in the hospital where the PRHO year will be spent. Multi-disciplinary teaching occurs between the medical and nursing schools for ethics and between the medical and midwifery schools for some parts of the Phase II reproduction, growth and development block. Teaching at Dundee has recently been rated excellent by the Scottish Higher Education Funding Council and well thought of in GMC assessments.

Traditional finals have been replaced with short exams and portfolio assessment. Phase exams are made up of MCQ-type and problem-based questions and an Objective Structured Clinical Exam (OSCE).

Course details

Course length	● 5 years
Total number of medical undergraduates	● 750
Male/Female ratio	● 45:55

Admission procedure

Average A level requirements	● ABB
Average Scottish Higher requirements	● AAABB
Number of applicants (Sept 2000 entry)	● 1250
Proportion of applicants interviewed	● 37%
Make up of interview panel	● Members of Faculty of Medicine
Months interviews held	● November–March
Number admitted (Sept 2000 entry)	● 154
Proposed entry size for 2001	● 154
Proportion of overseas students	● 7.5%
Proportion of mature students	● 16% (includes graduate entrants)
Faculty's view of taking a gap year	● Acceptable
Proportion taking Intercalated Hons	● 6%
Possibility of direct entrance to clinical phase	● None

Finances

Tuition fees per year	● £1050
Fees for self-funding students	● £1050
Fees for graduates	● £1050
Fees for overseas students	● £10 700 p.a. (pre-clinical) £17 000 p.a. (clinical)
Assistance for elective funding	● Yes – competitively every year some 20 awards are made £1000 max–£200 min
Assistance for travel to attachments	● No – responsibility of LEA
Access and hardship funds	● Yes – both grants and loans available within Medical School

Average cost of living

Weekly rent	● Halls £68 Private £50
Pint of lager	● Union Bar £1 City Centre pub £1+
Cinema	● £3 student night, £4 other 3 Multiplex approximately 30 Screens
Nightclub	● £2.50 Large selection offering all tastes in music/dance and entertainment

Dundee

Placements outside the university   In the second and third year teaching is mostly local: Ninewells and Kings Cross Hospital are within about 3 miles of each other. Some orthopaedics teaching is at Perth Royal Infirmary, 20 miles away. In the fourth and fifth year you get a chance to travel around the UK and see how other hospitals work: up to 5 months of the fourth year can be spent away from Dundee on outblocks. Placements with DGHs and GPs are set up around the UK from the Highlands and Islands to Cornwall, but mainly in Scotland. Hospital accommodation/living allowances are available.

Honours year   Honours year medical (and dental) students are invited by faculty to take an intercalated BMSc. Subjects typically include medical/social sciences, but BAs can also be taken.

Elective study/SSMs   Over 42 SSMs are advertised on the Medical School website, or you can design your own – overseas options are available. Staff are very supportive of individually designed SSMs happening in their clinics/labs. Fifth year kicks off with a 7 week elective (9 weeks if you tack on your 2 week vacation!). It's up to you to organise your own programme. Information and help regarding funding is widely available.

Course organisation   Each systems block, which typically lasts 4 weeks, has a Systems Convenor. You get a new study guide at the beginning of each block. Students are requested to give formal feedback regarding quality of teaching to the Medical School. You choose your own special study modules and outblock placements in the fourth year.

PRHO year   The Tayside region is now part of the all Scotland matching scheme for house jobs. During your fifth year you have the opportunity to spend a month shadowing both your medicine and surgery house jobs where you will be actually working.

The learning environment

The first year is based at the main campus, in the city centre. Years 2–5 are hospital based. Ninewells is about 3 miles from the town and main campus on the Firth of Tay. Wards have spectacular river views. Many students walk (30 minutes), bike or drive in, but numerous buses run right to the front door (fare 85p). Car parks are available: 60p for student parking, or £1 to be very close to the front door!

Library facilities   Year 1 books are housed in the newly extended library on the main campus. Year 1–5 books are housed at Ninewells Library. Opening hours are Monday to Friday 9 a.m.–10 p.m.; Saturday and Sunday 9 a.m.–6 p.m. There is good availability of reference books, but be prepared to reserve some books in advance.

Computer facilities   There is extensive computer access at both Ninewells (open 8 a.m.–11 p.m. all week) and the main campus. Facilities include computer assisted learning (CAL) tutorials, microbiology lab summaries, MCQs, MRI/CT/X-ray imaging, revision sessions, email and internet. Classes are laid on in IT skills for the nervous!

Clinical skills laboratory   The purpose-built Clinical Skills Centre opened in 1997. It provides multi-professional and multi-disciplinary teaching to small groups in areas such as communication and history taking; professional attitudes and ethics; physical examination and lab skills, diagnostics and therapeutics; and resuscitation. The Centre is open 9 a.m.–5 p.m. for teaching and drop-in revision sessions. The clinical and administrative staff are extremely supportive and proactive, and run a book-in service for revising clinical skills. Facilities include access to anatomical models and mannequins; diagnostic, therapeutic and resuscitation equipment; videos; simulated and real patients; and telemedicine links. Typical clinical skills sessions are generally good fun, last 2 hours and allow students to develop confidence and competence in clinical skills before going on to the wards.

Teaching hospitals   The staff tend to be friendly, approachable and supportive. They really do make an effort to ensure that students get the extra clinical training, core knowledge and time for small group work required by the new curriculum.

Student friendliness and support   A new staff-student leisure facility at Ninewells was completed in 1998, and a house officer facility was completed in 1996. The School of Nursing and Midwifery joined the Faculty of Medicine and Dentistry in 1997. Ninewells has its own swimming pool, squash courts, tennis courts and Medical Centre Bar. Each student is assigned a personal and academic tutor. There is a Special Needs Co-ordinator, based at Student Welfare on the main campus. The Dean is very approachable and student friendly, and operates an open-door policy. Likewise, lecturers and clinicians are approachable, and typically put a lot of work into designing and teaching each systems block. All medical freshers are sent a student-produced Student Survival Guide which covers academics, social, sport, local transport, etc. The students run a Senior-Junior scheme. There is also a very active Medical Students Council which regularly attends faculty meetings to voice student opinion. A good indicator of staff-student relations is the number of staff who regularly attend Year Club and hospital balls. The Medical School has good wheelchair access.

Student life

Accommodation   There are two halls on campus. Belmont is a large 1960s catered hall of residence next to the Union, the Sports Centre, and the Library. Airlie is a smaller self-catering hall on the other side of the Union and the Library. Peterson House and Seabraes Flats are a 1 minute stumble from campus. They are both self catering and the latter was built in 1996, with flats with en-suite bathrooms, etc. The West Park Centre is half-way between the town and Ninewells in the leafy west end of Dundee and offers both catered and self-catering halls. This accommodation was also built in 1996, and has self-contained flats with phones, en-suite bathrooms, colour TVs and computer links to the university internet. Most first years live in hall. Private accommodation costs £40–£50 per week and standards are pretty good.

Entertainment and societies   Dundee University Medical Society (DUMS) sponsors Freshers Week events, and puts on bashes throughout the year. Each year has its own Year Club to put on events – for example Freshers Week and end of year balls, fancy dress parties, nights out, pub golf and slave auctions – to raise money for charity. Ceilidhs (Scottish dancing) are very popular and are a great ice-breaker. Lessons are given for the uninitiated. Each Year Club organises a Half-way Dinner (weekend away with ball, etc.) guess when – half-way through the course! The Student Union building has been refurbished and hosts packed-out club nights through the week.

Local pubs abound, and the beer is cheap. The Cooler Nightclub is popular, and has won Scottish club scene awards. The Dundee Rep Theatre is active nationally, and hosts plays, musicals and jazz festivals.

The new Arts Centre just opened last year and provides two screens for "arthouse" films, a large art gallery, café and wine bar all right beside the university. The Stacks Leisure Complex offers a £3 student night on Mondays. The ABC in town offers cheap films. The Duncan of Jordanstone Art School is part of the main campus and their Summer Final Year Show is always a sell-out.

Sports facilities   The newly extended Sports Centre now boasts the largest university indoor facilities in Scotland. Outdoor pitches are based at the scenic and windy Riverside Drive. The university has a very active and varied sports scene, with a good level of competition in both Scottish and British university competitions. The Medical School has its own mixed teams in hockey, basketball and volleyball. There are also football, rugby and netball teams. Medics often play for both the Medical School and the university, with the Medical School teams being a little less competitive in spirit than the Dundee University clubs. A number of non-competitive trips and activities are open to all students and staff, such as sailing, hill walking, climbing, ceilidh lessons, skiing, outdoor pursuit weekends. Everybody is welcome, from beginners to the experienced.

City and surrounds   Dundee is Scotland's fourth largest city and has a beautiful location on the Firth of Tay. Local sights include the riverside itself, the neighbouring seaside town of Broughty Ferry with its sandy beaches, castle, shops and pubs; Tentsmuir Forest Park and beaches; Carnoustie; St Andrews (15 miles away); numerous golf courses and fantastic sunsets. As well as being spectacular, the countryside offers skiing, hill walking, climbing and numerous water sports. Dundee is not a cosmopolitan shopping centre, but the council is working to improve the city. The centre has been pedestrianised, the 1960s shopping centre is being demolished and replaced with something that is hopefully easier on the eye, and a number of new small shops, cafés, bars and clubs have opened over the past 12 months. There is constant building and renovation work in the town. Glasgow, Edinburgh and Aberdeen are all within reach for a weekend, from a 1–1½ hour drive/train journey away.

The five BEST things about Dundee Medical School

- Good teaching on a modern course.
- Good social life based around the Medsoc and a friendly bunch of staff and students means that you can always find something to do.
- Dundee is a cheap place to live.
- The Clinical Skills Centre is excellent.
- Dundee is surrounded by beautiful countryside, with access to skiing, hill walking and watersports.

The five WORST things about Dundee Medical School

- It can take some time to get used to the local accent.
- During the 4th and 5th year the attachments mean that the year group does not meet up very often.
- Dundee is not a great centre for shopping.
- Whilst having enough facilities for all normal needs, Dundee is not the most cosmopolitan or attractive city – unless you like bingo.
- It does get cold and windy here.

Further information

Admissions: Information Centre
Admissions and Student Recruitment
2 Airlie Place
The University of Dundee
Nethergate
DUNDEE DD1 4HN
Tel: 01382 344160
Fax: 01382 348150

East Anglia

Email: admissions@uea.ac.uk
www: http://www.uea.ac.uk

One of two new medical schools to be created will be at the University of East Anglia (UEA) in Norwich. The following is a statement from the School:

School of Medicine

MB/BS Medicine

A brand new Medical School is being launched at UEA and will offer an innovative five-year degree programme starting in September 2002. We are committed to equipping our students with an appropriate range of skills and knowledge for medical practice in the 21st century and our curriculum reflects the latest developments in medical education. Initially there will be 110 places.

Admissions policy

Successful applications will usually need to have three A levels (typical offer AAB) or their equivalent if offering other qualifications. In particular, we expect candidates to demonstrate a sound knowledge of biological sciences (grade A at A level, or equivalent), as well as academic attainment and potential in a range of scientific or other subjects. Normally at least five subjects, including both English and Mathematics, should have been passed at Grade A or B at GCSE or its equivalent.

We welcome applications from graduates in any subject and from other mature candidates with qualifications differing from those of school leavers. Entry from approved Access courses will be particularly encouraged.

No offer will be made without an interview, during which reasons for wishing to study medicine will be explored. Satisfactory medical and police screening will be required.

Curriculum

As a new Medical School we are working closely with the General Medical Council, which is responsible for validating our programme. Some details may change as our plans develop, but core principles are as follows.

In our curriculum, relevant skills and knowledge – including clinical and life sciences, as well as socio-economic aspects (eg sociology, psychology, epidemiology, management, health economics, law and ethics) – will be studied in relation to particular clinical conditions and the ways in which patients display them to doctors. These clinical presentations are grouped into units of learning based upon body systems (e.g. circulation).

To ensure a proper integration between theory and practice, students will spend a substantial part of each year gaining clinical experience with patients, both in secondary care (eg hospitals) and primary care (i.e. with GPs in health centres throughout the area). Where appropriate, experience of tertiary care (i.e. specialist centres) will also be provided. The nature and extent of this integration is one the most distinctive features of our course.

As well as covering the core medical curriculum, students will have the opportunity throughout to study areas of special interest in more depth and, in later years, to take some courses in subjects outside medicine. In the fourth year there is an 'elective' clinical placement period of 8 weeks in which each student chooses the type and location of clinical experience.

Our programme offers a variety of formats and experiences to encourage student learning. Whole-class discussions, lectures, seminars – and, especially, small-group sessions – are featured in our timetable. Clinical, communication and IT skills are taught throughout the course. Ample time is permitted for independent study. At the end of each of the first four years there is an integrative period to enable consolidation of the course to date. A similar period at the end of the final year is specifically set aside as preparation for employment as Pre-registration House Officers after graduation.

Assessment is on a unit-by-unit basis: there are no final examinations. Arrangements include multiple choice questionnaires; portfolios, presentations and projects; "advanced notice" questions in which research answers need to be presented under examination conditions; and Objective Structured Clinical Examinations (OSCEs).

Academic years (excluding breaks) are provisionally 32 weeks for Year 1, 39 weeks for each of Years 2 – 4 and 33 weeks for Year 5.

After graduation

As far as practicable, UEA graduates will be employed as PRHOs by our NHS partners (in hospitals and in general practice), so that we can offer mentoring and postgraduate study during the year.

Facilities

A new, specially-designed building is being constructed for the Medical School at UEA. In addition, the School will make extensive use of the leading-edge facilities at the new Norfolk and Norwich Hospital – which is very close to the University campus – as well as other hospitals, GP premises and health care facilities across the region.

Residential accommodation on UEA's attractive campus is guaranteed to first year students (en-suite options available). There is good private-sector provision of houses, flats and bed-sits in Norwich, a city which – while big enough to offer all the facilities of a major commercial and cultural centre – still manages to be a friendly, easy-going and safe place to live.

Further information

The Admissions Office
School of Medicine
University of East Anglia
Tel: 01603 593061
Fax: 01603 593752
Email: med.admiss@uea.ac.uk

Edinburgh

Although one of the oldest medical schools, Edinburgh has shed the traditional pre-clinical/clinical course in favour of a new integrated curriculum that started in October 1998. With a strong research tradition (reflected by 40% of students taking an intercalated BSc), Edinburgh seems to attract high academic achievers and a lot of students from England and Northern Ireland. The Medical School is situated centrally, which means that you mix well with other students and feel a real part of the university and the city itself – a compact, yet varied, centre to escape into.

The course

The new curriculum starts with the normal function of the body (year 1), and builds through disease processes (year 2) and clinical systems (year 3), to clinical contexts (years 4 and 5), whilst on attachment in GP practices, teaching hospitals and DGHs. It is taught in a fully integrated fashion, with themes of clinical skills and communication skills running across all 5 years. Although there is some clinical involvement in the early years (particularly through general practice), the bulk of clinical placements are in years 3-5.

Teaching and assessment   The general trend is towards lectures and tutorials for the whole year in the first couple of years, with formalised en-masse teaching being replaced by ward-based teaching later on in the course. Although there are some problem-based tutorials, most of the teaching is formal. Anatomy is taught by prosection and computer-assisted learning, and whilst animal tissue is used in some practicals, this is not compulsory. Exams have traditionally been at the end of each term and have counted for 100%. There is an increasing amount of continuous and modular assessment in the new curriculum.

Placements outside the university   In the second year time is spent in local GP practices learning clinical skills. In years 4 and 5, a significant amount of time is spent on 4-week blocks in peripheral hospitals up to 80 miles from Edinburgh. There are normally at least two students on the placement, and accommodation is provided free of charge. As there are fewer students you get much more involved in the team, and the teaching is generally as good (if not better) than the teaching in the central teaching hospitals. However, transport can often be difficult if you don't have a car.

Honours year   At Edinburgh there is a well-established honours year programme. 40% of the year group intercalates so you will quickly reintegrate when you rejoin the mainstream medicine course.

Elective study/SSMs   The elective takes place in either the 4th or 5th year and lasts 2½ months. The faculty is totally flexible about what you do – you can basically go anywhere and do anything medically related. There are also

65

several periods for Special Study Modules, starting in small groups in the 1st and 2nd years and leading to an independent research project for 14 weeks in the 4th year. This is a great opportunity to do your own ground-breaking research: one group of students organised an international high altitude research expedition in their SSM this year.

Course details

Course length	● 5 years
Total number of medical undergraduates	● c. 1150
Male/Female ratio	● n/a

Admission procedure

Average A level requirements	● AAB (Chemistry + 2 of Biology/Maths/Physics or Chemistry, Biology + other)
Average Scottish Higher requirements	● AAAAB (Chemistry + 2 of Biology/Physics/Maths)
Number of applicants (Sept 2001 entry)	● 2632
Proportion of applicants interviewed	● 1%
Make up of interview panel	● 2 members of admissions committee + Associate Dean
Months interviews held	● January–March
Number admitted (Sept 2001 entry)	● 220
Proposed entry size for 2001	● 220
Proportion of overseas students	● 4%
Proportion of mature students	● 3%
Faculty's view of taking a gap year	● Approved if it extends general education and experience
Proportion taking Intercalated Hons	● 35–40%
Possibility of direct entrance to clinical phase	● Yes

Finances

Tuition fees per year	● £1050
Fees for self-funding students	● Please check with Edinburgh
Fees for graduates	● Please check with Edinburgh
Fees for overseas students	● £9480 p.a. (pre-clinical) and £17 230 p.a. (clinical)
Assistance for elective funding	● Faculty gives some bursaries (up to £400 per student)
Assistance for travel to attachments	● No
Access and hardship funds	● Yes, administered centrally through the main university, and the Students Union gives short-term emergency loans

Average cost of living

Weekly rent	● Halls £84 Private £45–£55
Pint of lager	● Union Bar £1.20 City Centre pub £1.90
Cinema	● £2.50–£5
Nightclub	● Free to £12

Course organisation   Generally things run very smoothly, although at times there is a lack of communication between different limbs of the course. Sometimes clinical teachers don't turn up. The new course is centrally planned and executed, which will hopefully tighten things up.

PRHO year   Most people try to stay in Edinburgh for their house jobs, and the computer-matching scheme prioritises students' preferences over the consultants'. There is a shortage of jobs in the area, however, so there are some disappointments.

The learning environment

For the first 2 years medics are a real part of the university, with the Medical School centrally placed among the rest of the university in George Square. It is very handy for all the library facilities, unions and halls, as well as having the Royal Infirmary next door. The other teaching hospital is a short bus ride across town. This may all change in the future because a New Royal Infirmary is planned to open early in the next decade several miles outside town. It is not yet clear how much of the Medical School will remain on the university site and how much will move out, but it will certainly change the feel of things. In the last 3 years of the course, most time is spent in the hospitals and often away from Edinburgh, so medics can begin to lose touch with their student roots.

Library facilities   There is a dedicated medical library which gets well used, and is especially busy at exam times. Availability of recommended textbooks on short loan is generally good. It is open 9 a.m.–10 p.m. (Monday to Thursday), and until 5 p.m. on Friday and Saturday and 12–5 p.m. on Sunday afternoon. Holiday opening is until 7 p.m., including during the summer break when there are still clinical students working. Most DGHs also have small libraries.

Computer facilities   There is a dedicated lab in the Medical School of 90 pcs, with word processing, email, internet and specially designed computer-assisted learning available. The lab is open 24 hours via a swipe card, but it can get very busy during the day. Facilities in hospitals are very poor with no access to the university network, although this is set to improve.

Clinical skills laboratory   There are labs at both the main hospitals, which are used for clinical skills, but mainly for resuscitation training.

Teaching hospitals   The two main teaching hospitals are the Royal Infirmary right next to the Medical School, and the Western General, which is a 25 minute bus ride away (about 70p). Both hospitals have an atmosphere of pioneering, "cutting-edge" medicine and surgery. The facilities for students are adequate. There is a tremendous range of patients to learn from and ward groups are normally small (six or seven students in the 3rd year – but tending to get a bit bigger – and two students per ward in the 4th and 5th years). If you put the effort in you'll get a lot out of it.

Student friendliness and support   Faculty can seem a bit harsh and traditional when you first arrive. While each student has a Director of Studies responsible for monitoring his/her progress and providing pastoral care, this really acts as a safety net. Faculty tends to take a hands-off approach, which on one level gives you freedom and independence, but can leave you feeling like a small drop in a big ocean. However, if you have genuine difficulties then the Faculty is extremely helpful and genuinely flexible. The Faculty has good relations with the Medical Students Council and a comprehensive Student Handbook is published jointly every year.

Student life

Edinburgh, the city of festivals, is a great place to spend 5 years of your life. The university is centrally placed with the Medical School in the heart of the university. Although the capital of Scotland, Edinburgh has more than its fair share of English and overseas residents, so there is a very cosmopolitan atmosphere. For the first 2 years you really blend into mainstream student life, but the time-consuming clinical years mean that you gradually drift away from the main student body. There is a strong community spirit within each year group, and no shortage of medic societies, sports clubs and socialising.

Accommodation   Accommodation is guaranteed to first years, either in halls or flats, but demand for halls (which are a good standard) is greater than the places available. After the first year most students get a group together and rent a flat from a private landlord or the university. Many students also choose to take out a mortgage to buy their own flats, renting rooms to other students. An advantage of Edinburgh is that most of the student accommodation is very central for the university and the city, and almost invariably within 15-20 minutes walking distance. However, the cold winters do put up your heating bills.

Entertainment and societies   The Medical Students Council, Royal Medical Society (which has rooms open 24 hours to members) and each year's Final Year Club organise social events, talks and balls. There is also a medics choir and orchestra, an active Christian Medics group, and the Medical School magazine 2nd Opinion, which is now joined up with the other Scottish schools. Apart from traditional medic activities (various balls, plays, revue, academic families), most students find their own entertainment in the city itself rather than relying exclusively upon medical societies. The Union is one of the largest in the country, offers a good range of societies, and is an excellent venue. It does have lots of competition from the city itself.

Sports facilities   The Medics rugby team is well organised and successful, with a formidable reputation on and off the field. A mixed hockey team has recently been formed and what it lacks (sometimes) in skill it makes up for in character. There are various year football and badminton teams. Medics tend to play a more active part in the wider university sports scene rather than just staying within the Medical School. Most sportspeople who represent the Medical School will also play for the main university and/or local clubs.

City and surrounds   Edinburgh has the advantage of being a compact and generally safe city where everything is within walking distance. It is a lively cosmopolitan capital city with a good pub and club scene, theatres and cinemas, shopping, and a lot of tourist attractions. Although a huge tourist trap (especially during the Military Tattoo and the International Festival and Fringe in the summer), the tourists' and students' paths don't really cross. Between the three universities there is a large student population which is well catered for. Edinburgh has one of the highest concentrations of pubs in a city centre, and most are licensed to 1 a.m. (clubs open to 3 a.m.). Green space is found at the meadows and Holyrood Park. Both are excellent, with friendly football, rugby, hockey, American football, korfball matches, etc. Edinburgh is well connected for getting to most other parts of the UK and countryside, and the great outdoors is not too far away if you want to get away from it all for some fresh air.

The five BEST things about Edinburgh Medical School

- Edinburgh is a vibrant and lively university and city with excellent shopping, pubs and clubs. The new Scottish Parliament has added to the city's buzz.

- Edinburgh hosts a lot of innovative and world respected research projects in clinical medicine and surgery. You will be taught by some very big names!

- You can drink in pubs and restaurants 24 hours a day if you know how (and want to).

- Hospitals offer a good range of patients and pathology , and there is a lot of patient contact with them in the new course.

- The medical students have a very good collective spirit especially in the first 3 years, without being too cliquey.

The five WORST things about Edinburgh Medical School

- Large numbers of tourists, festival luvvies and the New Year Hogmanay invasion.

- The support network works well in a crisis, but you can feel a bit anonymous to the Faculty at other times.

- Peripheral attachments in the latter years mean that the year group doesn't meet up very often.

- Without a car, travelling to peripheral hospitals can be awkward.

- It gets very cold and windy in winter.

Further information

Undergraduate admissions: Faculty of Medicine
Medical School
Teviot Place
Edinburgh
EH8 9AG
Admissions Office: Tel: 0131 650 3187
Fax: 0131 650 6525

Email: medadmissions@pms.ac.uk
www: http://www.pms.ac.uk

Exeter and Plymouth-Peninsula

For the first time since the early seventies the government has announced the creation of new medical schools. One of the new institutions is the product of collaboration between the Universities of Exeter and Plymouth. The School is called the Peninsula Medical School. The following is a statement from the School.

The Peninsula Medical School will accept its first intake of 127 students in October 2002. The School is a joint venture between Exeter and Plymouth Universities in partnership with the NHS in the south west.

The first two years of study will take place at the two universities and, upon successful completion of that phase, will then continue for another two years in and around the teaching hospitals of Derriford in Plymouth, the Royal Cornwall Hospital in Truro and the Royal Devon and Exeter Hospital in Exeter. The fifth year, leading to graduation, will also include placements in hospitals in Torbay and Barnstaple as well as in general practice throughout the south west.

The Peninsula Medical School is one of two new medical schools announced by the government last year – the first in the UK since 1971 – which are designed to increase the number of doctors in the NHS. Both Exeter and Plymouth Universities have a strong track record of postgraduate medical training and research, and Plymouth also provides the nurse training for the south west, so teaching undergraduates is a natural development. The medical school will be the first in the south west, helping to meet a regional as well as a national need. The curriculum has been designed with the help of national experts very much in line with the most up to date thinking such as the General Medical Council's *Tomorrow's Doctors*. It aims to equip its graduates with the right skills and attitudes for the health service of the 21st century.

In particular:
- The student will receive an education in a research-rich environment which will emphasise the molecular basis of disease and the impact of the human genome project on medicine. The programme is designed to aid lifelong learning, reflective practice, and contribution to continuous quality improvement in the National Health Service.

- The course will be community-wide, reflecting the belief that doctors need to adopt a socially accountable approach to their work and to understand the human and societal impact of disease as well as the community context of contemporary healthcare provision.

Other important features of the course include education that is based upon the solution of problem cases, early contact with patients and acquisition of clinical skills. Head of the new medical school is Queen's Prize-winning diabetes expert, Professor John Tooke, who led the project team to success in the bid and has now been appointed Dean. He said:

"The Peninsula Medical School will be unique and special in several different ways. One of its aims is to broaden access to medical education by offering bursaries and encouraging applications from people from disadvantaged backgrounds and by enabling the direct entry of graduates from health-related disciplines who have at least two years post qualifying experience.

"Another is to establish a community-wide programme – rather than one that is based in a large, single teaching hospital. Through experiencing all facets of the NHS in hospitals, GP practices and in the community, students will be able to appreciate the importance of the multi-professional nature of modern health care and the essential integration of primary, secondary, diagnostic and management services.

"In addition, the programme will underline the importance of communication skills and the need for a doctor to understand – not only the nature of the disease itself - but also the personal impact of illness on individuals and their families."

For further information about the Peninsula Medical School and its curriculum see its website at: http://www.pms.ac.uk or call the School Administrator, Pat Bailey on 01752 764261.

For general information on studying at Exeter or Plymouth visit their websites: www.exeter.ac.uk and www.plymouth.ac.uk

c. 1200 students
Email: amp1v@clinmed.gla.ac.uk
www: http://www.gla.ac.uk

Glasgow

Glasgow is one of the longest established medical schools in Britain. In keeping with its reputation as a centre of excellence, it has radically updated its course in recent years to meet the demands of modern medicine. The new curriculum, introduced over five years ago, shifts the balance from spoon-fed learning to a more problem-based approach. Change and modernisation at the Medical School has been matched in other areas of the university, such as a well-equipped modern library and a gym and sports complex. In the unlikely event that you tire of the endless medical social functions, Glasgow has a social scene to rival any major city.

The course

Glasgow radically changed its curriculum in 1996. The course is now fully integrated, with students on the wards and clinical experience being provided from the outset. Information technology is taught and used from first year. The whole curriculum is student-centred and there is an emphasis on learning in small groups.

Teaching and assessment   Whole-class lectures only take place twice a week. The mainstay of the course is problem-based learning sessions. These involve groups of ten students, guided by a facilitator, tackling two medical scenarios each week. The traditional pre-clinical/clinical divide has been significantly eroded – patient contact and practical skills are now taught from week 1. Continuous assessment occurs every five–week block (in first and second year) via coursework, two 1 hour formal written exams are taken at the end of the first year. An Objective Structured Clinical Exam (OSCE) is also part of the assessment from the second year onwards. Years four and five are treated as a continuum, therefore there are no exams at the end of fourth year.

Placements outside the university   Peripheral attachments can take you to Paisley (8 miles) or as far as Dumfries (65 miles). However, there are many hospitals and general practices in the Greater Glasgow area and GP practices are likely to be local.

Honours year   There are both one and two year intercalated degree options. One year courses are available in clinical or science subjects and lead to a BMedSci (hons). The two year option is only available in science subjects. The intercalated degree courses start after year three.

Elective study/SSMs   Special Study Modules cover a wide range of subjects and constitute about 20% of the overall course time. Students choose from a list of options in the second year (there are no SSMs in first year) and then propose their own from third year onwards. Almost any topic can be proposed, including non-medical subjects such as French or Philosophy. SSMs can also be taken abroad in fourth and fifth years. There are two 4-week electives during the summers of the third and fourth year, which can also be spent abroad.

Course organisation   The course is well organised with friendly, approachable staff, who make themselves available to discuss any problems with the course. The faculty also continually monitor how the course is delivered (through questionnaires and staff–student committees) and try to respond to any issues raised by students.

Course details

Course length	● 5 years
Total number of medical undergraduates	● 1200
Male/Female ratio	● 2:3

Admission procedure

Average A level requirements	● AAB (at first attempt) in Chemistry and at least one of Biology/Maths/Physics (with the other two at GCSE)
Average Scottish Higher requirements	● AAAB in year 5 Chemistry and Biology plus one of Maths/Physics
Number of applicants (Sept 2000 entry)	● 1159
Proportion of applicants interviewed	● 58%
Make up of interview panel	● Two doctors and a member of admissions staff
Months interviews held	● November–March
Number admitted (Sept 2000 entry)	● 239
Proposed entry size for 2001	● Approximately the same
Proportion of overseas students	● 7%
Proportion of mature students	● Varies by year, no quota
Faculty's view of taking a gap year	● Acceptable so long as the year is used constructively
Proportion taking Intercalated Hons	● Approximately 50% (mainly for 1 year course)
Possibility of direct entrance to clinical phase	● No

Finances

Tuition fees per year	● £1050
Fees for self-funding students	● £1050
Fees for graduates	● £1050
Fees for overseas students	● £13 960 (2000–01)
Assistance for elective funding	● Small amounts available from Faculty
Assistance for travel to attachments	● No
Access and hardship funds	● Some Access fund money available centrally

Average cost of living

Weekly rent	● Halls £40–£70 Private £50–£60
Pint of lager	● Union Bar £1.50 City Centre pub £2.20
Cinema	● £3–£4
Nightclub	● Free–£15 (depends where you want to go!)

PRHO year   Most graduates remain in the Greater Glasgow vicinity due to the wide choice of jobs available, high teaching standards, and high pass rates for postgraduate exams. Matching is now via the Scottish PRHO Matching Scheme.

The learning environment

Glasgow has a large, attractive university campus in the West End of the city, 2 miles from the centre. Six large teaching hospitals within the Glasgow area and 13 District General Hospitals (DGHs) provide the mainstay of the teaching. Lectures generally take place at a variety of venues on campus including the modern Western Infirmary Lecture Theatre and the West Medical Building. A new £10m medical school building is currently being built as part of the University's 550th Anniversary and is due to be completed ready for use in September 2002.

Library facilities   The main Library, with an excellent range of reference books and journals, is open until 9.30 p.m. on weekdays and during the day at weekends. Study facilities are available on campus (24 hour in Unions) and in all hospitals, some of which are open 24 hours. The new building will also have extensive library and computing facilities.

Computer facilities   There is good central provision of computers in the main Library, with over 300 PCs available. Another 100 PCs are currently available on campus for medical students only. Facilities are increasing and improving all the time, with about 20 PCs available for students in each of the main teaching hospitals, but most peripheral hospitals are not yet linked to the campus network.

Clinical skills laboratory   Students are taught clinical skills from year one and there are also facilities for first aid and basic/advanced resuscitation training. However these have restricted access. The clinical skills facilities are made freely available for revision in the run up to exams and facilities will further improve with the new building.

Teaching hospitals   The teaching hospitals used include the Glasgow Royal Infirmary, the Western Infirmary, Gartnavel and Stobhill Hospitals. The medical and nursing staff are approachable and friendly. Some of the DGHs used are some distance away, but accommodation is provided and the facilities are mostly OK. Groups of students number between five and eight. This drops to two per ward by the final year.

Student friendliness and support   Glasgow is renowned for its friendliness and the medical school is no exception. Each student is allocated an adviser of studies to offer advice and support, and most tutors are approachable. Med-Chir (the medics' own society) operates a "Mums and Dads" scheme for freshers (with second years acting as parents!) and Glasgow has the usual university counselling and welfare services. The Students Representative Council (SRC) is currently working to improve disabled access. Students at the University and especially the medical school come from all over the UK and the rest of the world, with over half of medics coming from outside Scotland.

Student life

Glasgow is Scotland's biggest city and is truly international, with a large city centre containing all that you would expect to find. The main university buildings are amongst Glasgow's landmarks, with beautiful architecture and real atmosphere. The Gilbert Scott tower is the highest point in the city. There is lots of student accommodation in flats in the West End close to the University, and near to great pubs, shops and a lively club scene.

Accommodation

Glasgow has a large number of students who live in the area, but it tries to guarantee accommodation to first year students moving to the city, and 35% of hall places are reserved to returning students. The vast majority of these places are in catered halls. The University has little control over private sector flats but there is an accommodation office to help you. Average rents are £65 per week for full board in halls, £40 (plus bills) per week, for a 52 week lease on a University flat, and £50–£60 (plus bills) per week for private flats.

Entertainment and societies

The Medico-Chirurgical Society (Med-Chir) is a educational and social society set up and run by medical students. This meets every Thursday with free beer and talks from a range of speakers on a variety of entertaining topics. They also arrange events including trips abroad, the annual ball, the annual revue, and a musical culture night. Each year has its own yearclub to organise club nights, ceilidhs, balls and raise money for a massive graduation ball. Unusually, Glasgow has two unions: Glasgow University Union (GUU) and Queen Margaret Union (QM), both with bars, clubs, catering facilities, and a regular programme of bands, balls and special events. The GUU has a debate chamber and Glasgow has won the World Debating Championships many times. All the usual, and some unusual, clubs and societies are run from the unions. These are available for students to join (you can see a selection of them on the University website).

Sports facilities

The sports centre at the heart of the campus has recently undergone a massive refurbishment programme. The facilities include a 25m pool, sauna, muscle conditioning/weights room, squash courts and sports hall. There is a variety of sports clubs on offer, from football and rugby through to swimming, squash, canoeing, and horse riding. The Med–Chir also has a medics football and rugby team.

City and surrounds

Glasgow was the 1999 City of Art and Design, which reflects its interesting architecture and design history. You are never short of something to do or see in Glasgow, from the well-established Kelvingrove Gallery, which houses one of the best art collections in the UK, to the new Museum of Modern Art. Glasgow also boasts some of the best shopping in Scotland (including over forty shops in the new city centre Buchanan Galleries) and a leading club/pub scene. Not for you? How about an old firm game: Glasgow has the two largest Scottish football teams and many first division rugby sides. The city hosts many international athletic events. If you want a change of scene, getting out of Glasgow is easy enough, with access to some of the best hill walking, climbing and skiing in the UK, a mere 1–2 hours away. Other Scottish cities are also close at hand, with Edinburgh and the new Parliament only 45 minutes away. Buses and trains leave every 15 minutes.

The five BEST things about Glasgow Medical School

- Problem based learning and integrated clinical teaching from the outset.
- Teaching by internationally acclaimed experts.
- West End location, close to pubs/clubs and with a great campus.
- Large number of teaching hospitals.
- Small group bedside teaching.

The five WORST things about Glasgow Medical School

- Large size of lecture classes (although there are only two a week).

- Weather's not the best!

- Little contact with students of other disciplines.

- A high proportion of medics are from the Glasgow area and this dilutes the mix of students to some extent.

- Some attachments can be a long way from Glasgow.

Further information

Admissions:　　Admissions Enquiries
Medical Faculty Office
11 Southpark Terrace
University of Glasgow
Glasgow
G12 8LG
Admissions enquiries Tel: 0141 330 6216
Fax: 0141 330 2776
Email: amp1v@clinmed.gla.ac.uk

1050 students
Email: prospectus@leeds.ac.uk
www: http://www.leeds.ac.uk

Leeds

The course at Leeds has undergone several changes recently and there is now a new integrated curriculum. Out with the old subject-based teaching of anatomy, biochemistry, physiology, etc., and in with a module-based integrated course. There is some clinically oriented teaching from year 1 and hospital-based teaching starts towards the end of year 2. Staff and departments have been receptive to any balanced criticisms and suggestions and this has generated a student friendly atmosphere. The students on the new course seem to be really enjoying it. The medical school has a real mix of students from up and down the country, as well as overseas and mature students. Medics here sometimes feel a little separated from the rest of the university. A strong feeling of togetherness within and between year groups and a good Medsoc and Medical Students Representative Committee (MSRC) make up for this.

The course

The course is systems based, including clinical experience from year 1. Modules include personal and professional development, biomedical sciences, transport, life cycles, nutrition and energy, and control and movement. For years 1 and 2 the academic year follows the rest of the university, but from year 3 the academic year becomes longer at the expense of holidays.

Teaching and assessment   Teaching is integrated with a mix of problem-solving exercises and lectures. The use of computer-based learning is increasing rapidly, with experiments, tutorials and practice test questions being placed on computer. Anatomy is still taught using dissection of human cadavers. Ward teaching can be variable. Assessments include essays, projects, and both essay and multiple choice exams.

Placements outside the university   A lot of district general hospitals are used, including Bradford, Hull, Scarborough and Wakefield. A few third year students spend a term in the Yorkshire Dales. In the fourth and fifth years, attachments can be even further afield. In the third year accommodation and transport is provided for residential attachments.

Honours year   A year long BSc can be taken, usually after the 2nd or 3rd year. Approximately 25% of students intercalate. This has increased in recent years and there is a range of scholarships available.

Elective study/SSMs   A 10 week elective is timetabled at the beginning of the fifth year. Many students travel overseas for this, and recent destinations have been Canada, Australia, Africa and Barbados. Special Study Modules start in the first year and feature throughout the course.

Leeds

Course organisation   Most of the course at present is well organised, and teaching usually happens as timetabled.

PRHO year   There is a matching scheme for house jobs, and most people stay in the area as there are plenty of jobs. Recently introduced 1 year house office posts covering general practice, paediatrics and anaesthetics are proving popular.

Course details

Course length	● 5 years
Total number of medical undergraduates	● c. 1050
Male/Female ratio	● 47:53

Admission procedure

Average A level requirements	● AAB (including Chemistry)
Average Scottish Higher requirements	● Please check with Leeds Medical School
Number of applicants (Sept 2000 entry)	● 3000
Proportion of applicants interviewed	● 15%
Make up of interview panel	● 2 consultants
Months interviews held	● November–March
Number admitted (Sept 2000 entry)	● 237
Proposed entry size for 2001	● 230
Proportion of overseas students	● 10%
Proportion of mature students	● 4%
Faculty's view of taking a gap year	● Positive if the year is used for work experience, voluntary service or travel
Proportion taking Intercalated Hons	● 25%
Possibility of direct entrance to clinical phase	● Very limited

Finances

Tuition fees per year	● £1050
Fees for self-funding students	● Please check with Leeds University
Fees for graduates	● Please check with Leeds University
Fees for overseas students	● £9000 p.a. (pre-clinical) and £16 915 p.a. (clinical)
Assistance for elective funding	● Awards and prizes available
Assistance for travel to attachments	● Some available in years 4 and 5
Access and hardship funds	● Access funds from Leeds University

Average cost of living

Weekly rent	● Halls £30–£93 Private £45–£50
Pint of lager	● Union Bar £1.20 City centre pub £1.90
Cinema	● £3–£5
Nightclub	● £3–£10

The learning environment

The Medical School lies on the very edge of Leeds University campus and is attached to the Leeds General Infirmary (one of the main teaching hospitals). The city centre is a 10 minute walk from the school, and buses run from the campus to all parts of Leeds.

Library facilities   The Medical Library is well equipped and stocked, and is open until 9 p.m. Monday to Thursday, 7 p.m. on Friday and 5 p.m. on Saturday.

Computer facilities   There is very good provision of computers throughout Leeds university, with 200 in the Medical School and about 50 in a cluster at St James' Hospital (Jimmy's). There is an IT course at the beginning of the first year to help improve computer literacy.

Clinical skills laboratory   There are clinical skills labs at St James' Hospital and at Leeds General Infirmary (LGI).

Teaching hospitals   Facilities in the teaching hospitals are generally okay. Lots of teaching happens at the two main Leeds' hospitals – Jimmy's and the LGI. The district general hospitals tend to be more friendly, with the staff seemingly more willing to teach, and good computer and library facilities.

Student friendliness and support   Levels of support at Leeds are generally good. A personal tutor scheme has been runnning for about three years and enables groups of about five students from different years to interact with the support of a member of staff. The Students Union and the University have counselling services.

Student life

Leeds is the fastest growing city in the UK outside London. The main city centre has all the shopping and nightlife your bank account could take, within a 10–15 minute walk from campus. Theatre, Opera North, museums and galleries cater for the culture vultures. Sport is big in Leeds, especially football, cricket, and rugby league.

Accommodation   All first years can live in university accommodation, either halls or flats. These can be pricey, but standards are generally good and this can be a good way to meet non-medics. In the second year most move out to back-to-back houses in Leeds 6 – Studentsville. Rent starts at about £45 per week but most pay a little more. Insurance is pricey, and burglary can be a problem. The locals can sometimes be a little anti-student, but your mates all live in the next street. There is help in finding accommodation available from the university.

Entertainment and societies   The Union has four bars including the biggest bar in Europe (allegedly). Medsoc is very active, with a ball early in November, and a dinner dance in March – not to be missed. They also organise ice-skating, quizzes, ballet trips and lots of general drinking nights – something for everyone. Medsoc is probably the most active society of the Union. The university also has a wide range of clubs and societies.

Sports facilities   Medics rugby, football, hockey, netball, cricket and racket games are all supported by MSRC. The university has a large sports centre, loads of gym equipment, aerobics classes, yoga, kickboxing, ju-jitsu, etc. The main university runs many sports teams as well.

City and surrounds   "Possibly the shopping capital of the north!" The city centre boasts the only Harvey Nichols outside London, and, with the many other shops, there is everything anyone could want. The Yorkshire Dales are a short bus journey away and a fantastic place to walk and get away from the hustle and bustle of life in Leeds. There are good road links and Leeds is on the Intercity rail network.

The five BEST things about Leeds Medical School

- The friendliness amongst medics between different years.

- The Leeds nightlife means there is always something for everyone to do.

- Very active medical student committees organising everything from balls to sports events.

- Proximity to the Dales – a city in the country!

- Leeds is a city on the up, and there is a definite buzz about the centre (and fantastic shopping).

The five WORST things about Leeds Medical School

- There are so many distractions from studying.

- Medics always seem to have exams when the rest of the university hasn't, and vice versa.

- Increased use of computers can lead to problems of access.

- Traffic, particularly at rush hour, and lots of road works are choking the city centre.

- Everywhere in Leeds is hilly!

Further information

Admissions: Admissions Office
School of Medicine
University of Leeds
Leeds
LS2 9JT
Admissions Tel: 0113 233 4362
Fax: 0113 233 4375

870 students
Email: admissions@le.ac.uk
www: http://www.le.ac.uk

Leicester (Leicester/Warwick)

Leicester is a young medical school, whose first medical students graduated in 1980. It is a friendly medical school with the teaching for Phase 1 on the university campus. The campus is next to Victoria Park about 10-15 minutes walk from the city centre. Most of the main halls are further out in one of the nicer areas of Leicester and they have beautiful gardens. The later phases of the course are based mainly at the Clinical Sciences Building. This is part of Leicester Royal Infirmary and near the city centre. The Union provides many a good night out, and there are also nights organised by MedSoc, including balls and doctors mess parties.

Stop press

The Universities of Leicester and Warwick have joined up to offer a 4 year medical degree course to graduates in biomedical sciences. The course started in 2000 with 64 students and the first intake has begun their studies at Warwick on an accelerated version of phase I of the Leicester 5 year degree programme. Upon successful completion of phase I students will join with the phase II programme at the University of Leicester.

Where possible we have given details for the Warwick course:

Course length	● 4 years
Total number of places	● 128 (2001 entry)
Admission requirements	● minimum 2.1 degree in a biomedical science
Number of applicants	● 491 (2000 entry)
Proportion of applicants interviewed	● 35%
Make-up of interview panel	● 1 academic or NHS Consultant and a final year medical student
Months interviews held	● November–February
Tuition fees per year	● £1050 (first year only)
Accommodation	● In postgraduate residences, guaranteed for the first year

Leicester

Statement from Leicester/Warwick Medical School:

"The Universities of Leicester and Warwick have become partners in a Medical School to provide an exciting opportunity for highly motivated graduates of Biomedical and Biological Sciences to become doctors in just four years. The new, graduate entry course is based upon the current highly successful 5 year curriculum in Leicester which was awarded 23 points out of 24 by the independent Quality Assurance Agency. The combination with Warwick's impressive record of teaching and research quality ensures that the new venture will provide an unrivalled learning environment for students to develop the knowledge, skills and attitudes to practice medicine. Like the five year curriculum, the new course is in two phases, Phase I and Phase II. All learning takes place in an obvious clinical context. For the new course Phase I has been shortened from $2^1/2$ years to $1^1/2$, by giving credit for prior learning. Phase II is wholly clinical and is identical in the two courses.

The overall aim of the Medical School is to prepare new doctors to meet the challenges of future health care delivery. Our graduates will take forward knowledge, skills, attitudes and values that will prepare them for the inevitable changes in practice that will come in the future. We place such emphasis on appropriate attitudes to medical practice that you will be required on graduation to affirm the Declaration of Geneva.

Dr W. Montague
Graduate Entry Coordinator

Further information:
Dr W Montague
Graduate Entry Co-ordinator
The Faculty Office
Leicester Warwick Medical School
Maurice Shock Building
PO Box 138
Leicester, LE1 9HN
Tel: 0116 2231452   http://www.lwms.ac.uk

The course

In common with most other medical schools, Leicester has largely done away with the traditional pre-clinical/clinical divide. The course is now separated into two phases, each lasting $2^1/2$ years. Phase I is taught in the Medical Sciences Building and is based on tutorials and lectures. There is, however, an introduction to clinical skills and you are let loose on wards in November of the second year. Anatomy is taught using dissection and prosections. There is also a clinical applications module to be completed in the third year on a disease of your choice. Phase II is mainly clinical, with ward teaching in different specialties, and includes an elective period. Progression between the two phases is subject to passing examinations.

Teaching and assessment
For Phase I teaching you are placed in a group of eight for tutorial work and will remain with this group throughout the phase. Examinations are mainly written short-answer questions or assessed essays; there are vivas for borderline passes or "excellents". Phase II teaching is on the wards, but it is backed by some lectures (an academic half-day per week). You will be with a clinical partner of your choice. Attendance is registered and contributes to passing modules. There are twelve 8-week blocks which rotate through disciplines. For each block, the pair of clinical students are attached to two consultant teams, one from a sub-specialty and one more general. Assessment includes patient portfolios (case studies) and clinical skills (histories and examinations). Finals have a clinical component and written examinations.

Course Details

Course length	5 years
Total number of undergraduates	870
Male/Female ratio	40:60

Admission Procedure

Average A level requirements	AAB (Chemistry + at least one other Science)
Average Scottish Higher requirements	AAB (Chemistry + Biology). Must offer CSYS
Number of applicants (Sept 2000 entry)	2107
Proportion of applicants interviewed	50%
Make-up of interview panel	Academic + final year student
Months interviews held	Nov–March
Number admitted (Sept 2000 entry)	179
Proposed entry for 2002	180
Proportion of overseas students	7%
Proportion of mature students	9%
Faculty's view of taking a gap year	Encouraged
Proportion taking Intercalated Hons	5%
Possibility of direct entrance to clinical phase	Unlikely

Finances

Tuition fees per year	£1050
Fees for self-funding students	£1050 p.a.
Fees for graduates	£1050 p.a.
Fees for overseas students	£8625 p.a. (pre-clinical) £16 950 p.a. (clinical)
Assistance for elective funding	Bursary scheme+£250 loan
Assistance for travel to attachments	None
Access and hardship funds	Available

Average Cost of Living

Weekly rent	Halls £40–£70 Private £32–£40
Pint of lager	Union £1–£1.50 City Centre pub £1–£1.80
Cinema	£3–£3.50 (with NUS card)
Nightclub	Free–£5 (with NUS card)

Leicester

Placements outside the university Leicester has three teaching hospitals: Leicester Royal Infirmary, Leicester General and the Glenfield Hospital. In addition, district general hospitals are used in Kettering, Coventry, Nuneaton, Boston, Lincoln and Peterborough, and free accommodation is provided. GP attachments are in Leicester and the surrounding area, with the furthest GP attachment in Rugby.

Honours year   Any student wishing to do an Honours year is encouraged to do so. Honours degrees can be science based or clinical and there is a wide range of projects to choose from. The year is usually taken after the 2nd year, but can be done after the third.

Elective study/SSMs   All students have a 2 month elective module which can be carried out in the UK or abroad. Two Special Study Modules are done in Phase I. Science modules are available as well as other subject areas such as language modules.

Course organisation   The new course was introduced in 1994 and is now well established, with structured teaching and self-study sessions.

PRHO year   Most students stay in the Leicester area for this year. A list of posts is available from November of the 5th year and selection of jobs is completed by January. Most students will be allocated a 12 month rotation consisting of three 4-month posts. The matching scheme for these posts works on a combination of student and consultant choice. Where possible they are matched, but there are obviously disappointments.

The learning environment

Phase I is based on the university campus in the Medical Sciences Building (MSB), and Phase II is based in the Clinical Sciences Building (CSB/Robert Kilpatrick Building) at the Leicester Royal Infirmary (LRI). The LRI is only a 10 minute walk from the MSB, and everything is in reasonable proximity. Teaching also happens at the General and Glenfield Hospitals, which are a short bus ride or, for the energetic, a cycle ride away.

Library facilities   The main university library is on campus and near to the MSB. There are also libraries at the three main teaching hospitals, but the CSB library at the LRI is the main library used by medical students. The MSB and CSB Libraries open from 9 a.m. to 10 p.m. on weekdays. The hours are shorter on Saturday (9 a.m.–6 p.m.) and Sunday 3 p.m–9 p.m.

Computer facilities   There are computer facilities in the Main Library, Charles Wilson, New Building and MSB on the main campus, but you do have to queue sometimes. There are plenty of computers (mostly PCs) through which you can access the internet and email. Course work (case studies and essays) must be word processed.

Clinical skills laboratory   There is clinical skills training with volunteers and communication skills with actors in the 1st year. After that the patients are real!

Teaching hospitals   The main teaching hospitals are the LRI, Leicester General and the Glenfield. DGHs across the region also teach students, but only in Phase II.

Student friendliness and support   The faculty staff at the MSB are very approachable and supportive, and some individual tutors are particularly accessible to discuss problems, etc. Each hospital has a student facilitator to deal with student queries and problems. There is always a member of staff available (24 hours) if there are any major problems or emergencies, and also a special counselling service at Student Health for medical students. Leicester University has a counselling service and some welfare services are available from the Students Union. Most areas of the Medical School and university have standard disabled access facilities, such as ramps and lifts.

Student life

The city centre is about a 45 minute walk from halls, or 10–15 minutes from the university campus. There is a regular bus service between halls, the town centre and the university during term-time. A good range of cinemas, theatres, pubs, clubs, bars and shops manage to reflect the city's diverse ethnicity. There are plenty of restaurants, and curry lovers have a wide choice of eateries. Many top bands take in Leicester on tour at De Montford Hall and at De Montford University. Leicester manages to have all the facilities of a city and some of the homeliness and friendliness of a smaller town.

Accommodation University accommodation is available throughout the degree and some medical students stay in Putney House beyond the 1st year. In the 1st year it is popular, and advisable, to live in catered halls as there are loads of activities and great end of term balls and parties. Digby has one of the best summer balls in the country. Privately rented accommodation is inexpensive but variable in quality. It is best to shop around in advance for a good deal. A Union-run accommodation office can help you find places.

Entertainment and societies At the Students Union there are club nights every Wednesday, Thursday, Friday and some Saturdays. Private parties take place at the start of the week. The bar is open all day every weekday, and on Saturday and Sunday nights. Food can be bought during the day. There are popular clubs in town and late bars to suit all tastes. The MedSoc holds parties every term, as well as the Christmas and Annual Dinners. There is a large variety of university societies to choose from; some are a bit mad, but if you want to join a society you will be spoilt for choice.

Sports facilities The Medical School sports teams - hockey, rugby (girls and boys), football and netball - are not great, but they are improving. The university teams are good and there are plenty to choose from. There are sports fields, two sports halls, two gyms, where there are circuits and aerobic classes, and a race-track. There are plenty of swimming pools in town.

City and surrounds The city is reasonably small, but has recently been redeveloped and has all the shops you could want. If you have a car, the Leicestershire countryside is attractive and makes a pleasant escape from the city. There is Premier League football and rugby on the doorstep, and there is a buzz about the place.

The five BEST things about Leicester Medical School

- Friendly medical school; students are welcoming.

- Phase 1 faculty staff are very friendly and approachable. They offer a wide range of help, from support with work to trying to help stressed or upset students.

- Leicester is easily accessible by train (Midland Mainline) and by road (M1).

- Great improvement in Leicester's nightlife in recent years, with many new bars, clubs and restaurants for varying tastes.

- Plenty of curry.

The five WORST things about Leicester Medical School

- Location of placements can present you with travel problems.

- MedSoc communication with the clinical years is poor due to the course structure and poor Phase I and Phase II relationships.

- Phase II students are spread about the region.

- Not near the sea. In fact Leicester is about as far from it as you can be.

- Too much curry!

Further information

Admissions: Admissions and Student Recruitment Office
Leicester University
University Road
Leicester
LE1 7RH
General admission enquiries Tel: 0116 252 2295
Fax: 0116 252 2447

Liverpool

In 1996 Liverpool Medical School introduced a brand new curriculum, in accordance with GMC guidelines. So far it is proving to be a success. This year all students at Liverpool are studying the new course, and in August 2001 the new house officers will be the first PBL students to qualify at Liverpool. Liverpool Medical School is growing in size, with 1000 undergraduates, but a strong Medical Students Society ensures there's always a friendly face around. Combine all this with one of the most vibrant cities in the UK makes for 5 years you are guaranteed not to forget!

The course

After extensive planning, a new problem-based learning (PBL) curriculum was introduced 5 years ago. Since its introduction course subjects are no longer taught in lecture theatres day in, day out: instead, different areas of medicine are presented to students as problems. Students discuss the issues and formulate learning objectives in small groups with tutor guidance. They then go away and research the information for themselves. From the beginning of the second year, an increasing proportion of time is spent on hospital and community attachments. Studies follow the human life cycle, from conception and birth, through adulthood and into old age.

Teaching and assessment   The new course contains little in the way of formal teaching. The few plenaries (lectures) that are given are designed to provide an overview only of each problem. It is then up to the student to find out further details from the other resources available. Alongside library work, students have formal training in clinical and communication skills. Anatomy is demonstrated using models and prosections. IT (information technology) has an ever increasing role, with various computer-based learning packages available. Assessment is continuous, designed so that everything you learn (including practical skills acquired) will be recognised and recorded. Most examination is by self-assessment questions at the end of each module, and formal exams occur in the first, third and fourth years. There are no exams in the final year! The final year is spent shadowing house officers in various specialities to prepare students for the realities of the house job.

Placements outside the university   In the first year, all teaching is done in the university. From the second year onwards, more time is spent on placements. For example on a typical 2 week module in the second year, one day is spent in a local GP practice and 2 days are spent either in a relevant community attachment, or at one of the hospitals. Placements are mainly within or near to Liverpool (Wirral, Southport, Warrington, Halton, etc.) but some are further away, such as Rhyl (North Wales) and Chester.

Honours year   It is possible to study for an intercalated degree at the end of the fourth year. Subjects available include Anatomy, Biochemistry, Cell Biology, Pharmacology, Physiology and Psychology. Some students study for an intercalated degree at another university and then return to complete the medical course at Liverpool. Limited funding is available to some students wishing to study for an Honours year.

Elective study/SSMs   The formal medical elective occurs in the third year, for 6 weeks. Six special study modules, each lasting 4 weeks, are spread through the 5 year course. Topics from any specialty can be chosen and an essay must be completed for each module.

Course details

Course length	● 5 years
Total number of medical undergraduates	● 1000
Male/Female ratio	● 40:60

Admission procedure

Average A level requirements	● AAB – Chemistry plus at least one other Science
Average Scottish Higher requirements	● AAABB – including Chemistry, Biology, Maths, Physics. English must have been passed at GCSE O level or SG level. 2 CSYS including Chemistry
Number of applicants (Sept 2000 entry)	● 1700
Proportion of applicants interviewed	● 56%
Make up of interview panel	● 2 senior clinical and academic staff
Months interviews held	● November–March
Number admitted (Sept 2000 entry)	● c. 215
Proposed entry size for 2001	● 268
Proportion of overseas students	● 15%
Proportion of mature students	● 15%
Faculty's view of taking a gap year	● Encouraged as long as the year has broad educational benefit
Proportion taking Intercalated Hons	● 10%
Possibility of direct entrance to clinical phase	● No

Finances

Tuition fees per year	● £1050
Fees for self-funding students	● Please check with Liverpool
Fees for graduates	● Please check with Liverpool
Fees for overseas students	● £13 150 p.a. (pre-clinical) and £16 800 p.a. (clinical)
Assistance for elective funding	● c. £12 000 p.a. to be divided on merit between student applicants
Assistance for travel to attachments	● None
Access and hardship funds	● Any full time UK student can apply for hardship awards but there are no guaranteed funds

Average cost of living

Weekly rent	● Halls £48–£76 Private £37–£60
Pint of lager	● Union Bar £1+ City Centre pub £1.80
Cinema	● £3+
Nightclub	● Free–£12

A new addition to the course is the SAMP– selective in advanced medical practice. This is a placement during the final year spent in a specialty chosen by the student.

Two exchange schemes – Socrates and Erasmus – allow students to study at a participating European medical school for a period of 16 weeks during Phase 3 of their course. Current exchanges are set up with schools in France, Germany, Holland and Sweden. The scheme has recently been expanded to include Eastern European countries.

Course organisation   Liverpool has offered a PBL course for the past 5 years. The experience of students who have already begun the new course has highlighted some of the organisational problems that inevitably occur when a syllabus changes. Communication between staff and students at Liverpool is good, and many of the early problems have been ironed out.

PRHO year   Applications for house jobs are made in the fourth year. The vast majority of students get their first job in the Mersey area, so the sense of community built up as students is retained after you qualify. The SHOs who teach you are often familiar faces from the medical school.

The learning environment

Liverpool University was the original redbrick university. The campus dominates a large area adjacent to the city centre and between the two cathedrals. The University Hospital is right next to the university campus, and the Medical School is well placed near to all the main university and hospital departments. The student body mixes well with the junior doctors at the hospital through Liverpool Medical Students Society (LMSS) meetings.

Library facilities   A short loan system operates for the books most in demand. The library is open until 9.30 p.m. most weekdays. Opening hours are more restricted at weekends and outside the main university terms, which differ from the medical school terms. All hospitals have their own libraries and borrowing arrangements for students vary.

Computer facilities   The university has 24 hour computer facilities available for students, with free use of email and the internet.

Clinical skills laboratory   One of the real highlights of the new course has been the introduction of the clinical skills lab, where students are able to master a whole range of practical doctoring skills, from taking blood and suturing wounds to giving advanced CPR. There are weekly classes in the first year, with a clinical skills exam at the end. Most students agree it is the best part of the week.

Teaching hospitals   The medical school is part of a large teaching hospital. The Royal Liverpool University Hospital. Also within the city centre is the Liverpool Women's Hospital, which has 200+ beds. Liverpool has its share of regional specialist centres, including Broadgreen Hospital and Alder Hey Children's Hospital are in the suburbs.

Student friendliness and support   Students generally mix well and there are good inter-relations within and between years. There is a long-standing mentoring system set up by the LMSS, so that each first year student is paired with a second or third year. In recent years Liverpool has enjoyed a very constructive and student-friendly atmosphere within the Faculty. The Students Union has the standard welfare and counselling services.

Student life

Liverpool offers an excellent welcome to students. It is a proud, yet warm city with its world famous accent, sense of humour, two cathedrals, football teams and maritime history. It was once the biggest port in the British Empire. Having fallen on hard times in the 70s and 80s, Liverpool is now very much on the up! Many students, from all courses, stay in the area after graduation. The Medical School and the student residential areas are well placed for all the attractions, and are adjacent to the many parks within the city. There is crime about but a common-sense approach will ensure that the good times aren't spoilt.

Accommodation   Most people only live in university accommodation for their first year. This is a good opportunity to meet other students from outside the Medical School, but university accommodation is more expensive than renting privately. There is a wide variation in the standard of private accommodation, but there is plenty of choice. The university has no input into regulating the private sector, but the accommodation office can offer advice.

Entertainment and societies   LMSS has weekly meetings with guest speakers. There are regular balls, dinners and social parties, as well as the medics' own orchestra, choir, sports teams, play and Christmas revue. The university also offers a wide range of different societies. LMSS has its own website at www.LMSS.org.

Sports facilities   The Medical Society has football, rugby, hockey, netball, basketball, squash, badminton, cricket and swimming teams. Recent additions to the sports teams include Chinese Martial Arts and a celebrated Tiddlywinks team! The university has all these and more! There are plenty of facilities.

City and surrounds   Liverpool has an excellent social side – every food taste catered for, excellent pubs, several cinemas, sports complexes, and nightclubs of all hues, from 70s clubs to Cream. It is also the home of two great football teams (Liverpool and Tranmere Rovers), one other (Everton) the world's most famous horse race, the Grand National at Aintree. (Oh, have we mentioned the Beatles yet?) The city is only a short distance from Manchester, North Wales, Chester and the Lake District.

The five BEST things about Liverpool Medical School

- The PBL course is self-directed and self-motivated, and allows you to adapt your learning to your pace.
- Students have a real say in the course at Liverpool, and course organisers are receptive to their suggestions.
- Liverpool medics students spend their time learning how to deal with real patients, not learning the Kreb's cycle.
- Liverpool is a relatively cheap city to live in.
- The main university teaching hospital has one of the largest accident and emergency departments in Europe.

The five WORST things about Liverpool Medical School

- The necessary approach to course work at Liverpool can be very different from A level studies; the PBL course is not for people who want to be spoon fed in lectures.
- Hospital placements can be some distance from Liverpool, and travelling by public transport can be time consuming and expensive.

- Anatomy is only taught through prosections, i.e. Blue Peter style "here's one we cut up earlier".

- University facilities are available during university term dates. Outside these 'normal term times', facilities, such as the library, are operated on restricted 'vacation hours'.

- The social life within the medical school can be so good that sometimes it is difficult to get to know students from other courses!

Further information

Admissions Administrator: Faculty of Medicine
1st floor Duncan Building,
Daulby Street,
Liverpool
L69 3GA
Admissions Tel: 0151 709 7172
Fax: 0151 706 5667

1443 students
Email: ug.admissions@.ac.uk
www: http://www.man.ac.uk

Manchester (Keele)

Manchester is one of the largest medical schools in Europe and is situated in the heart of a busy cosmopolitan city with something for everyone. Medicine has been taught here for centuries. A new integrated curriculum was introduced in 1994 which involves a problem-based approach to training. Although a pre-clinical/clinical divide exists, the basic sciences are studied within a clinical framework. A huge emphasis is placed on self-directed learning, allowing students time to focus on the aspects of the course which interest them most in greater depth. Manchester is in a unique position in that students are joined in the 3rd year by an intake of students from St Andrews.

Stop press

The Universities of Manchester and Keele won funding to provide training and education for undergraduate medics from October 2000. Fifty places are available to students who will begin their training at Manchester and two years later move to Keele to complete their undergraduate training. The final three years will be spent in clinical training at Keele and the North Staffordshire Hospital and Combined Healthcare trust.

Where possible we have put the details for the Keele course below:

Proposed number of students	● 50 per year in collaboration with Manchester University Medical School
Course length	● 5 years but possible to include a BSc year or a first year for those without science A levels
Average A level requirements	● AAB
Average Scottish Higher requirements	● AAAAB (for entry to 6-year course only)
Expected proportion of applicants interviewed	● 60%
Make-up of interview panel	● Four interviewers – combination of consultants, general practitioners, bioscientists
Months interviews held	● Mid November–Early April
Expected proportion of mature entrants	● 10–15%
Faculty's view of taking a gap year	● Acceptable
Intercalated degree option	● Yes – Wide range of bio-science and medicine related subjects available (e.g. Ethics and Law, History of Medicine)

Tuition fees per year	• £1050 – maximum contribution from student – LEA pay remainder
Fees for self-funding students	• £1050
Fees for graduates	• £1050
Fees for overseas students	• £6800 years 1 and 2; £9000 years 3, 4, and 5
Assistance for elective funding	• Students can apply for bursaries
Assistance for travel to attachments	• None
Access and hardship funds	• Yes subject to eligibility rules
Average weekly rent	• Halls £35–£60 all self catering; (private) £35–£40 depending on letting period and type of accommodation.
Pint of lager	• Union Bar £1 before 10 p.m., £1.45 after 10 p.m.; City Centre pub £1.70–£1.80
Cinema	• Keele Film Society on campus offers weekly programme – tickets £2 Multi screen Odeon cinema at Festival Park, Hanley – £3.40, Warner Village – £3 (with union card) Stoke Film Theatre (Staffordshire University) tickets £2.50

The course

The course is 5 years long, with 2 years pre-clinical followed by 3 years clinical. The pre-clinical course is structured around weekly cases that are studied through a mixture of group discussion, practical anatomy and pathology labs, computer skills sessions, lecture theatre events, and personal study. The course is organised into four semesters, so that cases relate to the four themes of nutrition and metabolism, cardiorespiratory, fitness abilities and disabilities, and life cycles. Years 3 and 4 continue the case-based approach in a more clinical setting, and the four themes are repeated. Four days per week are spent in one of the big teaching hospitals, with one day per week spent in GP surgeries. The fifth year is residential and allows students to shadow house officers and gain practical experience to prepare them for their pre-registration house jobs. The fifth year includes an elective.

The European Option   At Manchester there is also the chance to do the "European Option" which is recognised in the degree awarded to those who successfully complete it. Students who have A level languages can study either French or German. Medical vocabulary is taught from year one and four months of year five are spent in France, Germany or Switzerland.

Teaching and assessment   First and second year teaching centres around a weekly case study with supplementary group discussions, lectures and practical sessions including microscopy, anatomy, tutorials using cadavers, basic clinical skills and computational skills. For those studying the "European Option" there are weekly lessons with homework set. The style of lesson will be familiar to A level language students but the standard is a little higher. In years 1 and 2 there are exams at the end of each semester. They comprise of two MCQs, two papers on a clinical case study, an exam requiring the interpretation of scientific prose into lay language, an OSCE and, unusually, a computer skills exam. At the end of each semester groups are assessed for communication skills and teamwork.

Statement from Keele University Medical School

Keele University is offering undergraduate medical education in partnership with Manchester University. You will be recruited through a joint selection process organised by Manchester and will spend your first two years in Manchester Medical School. After that, students are dispersed between four clinical teaching hospitals and the Keele students will come to North Staffordshire NHS Trust. This is a very busy hospital offering the full range of clinical services and an excellent place to gain clinical experience. Three miles from the hospital is Keele University which is based on a large attractive campus with restaurants, social and sports facilities as well as library and academic buildings. Year 3 students will be guaranteed accommodation on the University campus so that they can integrate quickly after their move from Manchester.

The structure of the course and the assessments are the same for Keele and Manchester students. Keele students can also take the 6 year option by incorporating a pre-first year (for those without science 'A' levels) or an intercalated BSc year.

The first students for Keele and North Staffordshire will arrive in October 2002 having started in Manchester in October 2000. Plans are progressing well to ensure that the additional academic and clinical facilities are in place. New staff will be recruited in the early part of 2002 as well as altering the responsibilities of existing staff. The local consultants and staff in partner district general hospitals are extremely enthusiastic about the new school and looking forward to the first group of students arriving.

Full contact address for admissions information:

Faculty of Health, Keele University on 01782 583902
or, Admissions Office on 01782 632343.
www.keele.ac.uk

Admissions and Recruitment Office:
Keele University
Staffordshire
ST5 5BG
Tel: 01782 584005/4010/3551
Fax: 01782 632343

Mrs E M Clark
Admissions Officer
Medical School
Stopford Building
Oxford Road
Manchester
M13 9PT
Tel: 0161 275 5025
Fax: 0161 275 5584
email address for enquiries/prospectus: aaa30@keele.ac.uk

Placements outside the university   In the third and fourth year, four days per week are spent at the Base hospital and one day at a GP surgery. However, it is worth noting that getting to and from placements can be difficult without a car. DGHs and Base hospitals are sometimes a distance from the main student areas and are not always served by frequent public transport. Year four students also spend seven weeks in a DGH when accommodation is provided. Students have the option of living in free hospital accommodation in their final year, as their placements may be some distance from Manchester. In the fifth year there are five main blocks, which are equal in length: one surgical, one medical one GP an elective and the consolidation period immediately prior to finals. These placements are chosen by the students and should include one teaching hospital and one DGH placement. Accommodation is free on placements. There is also a four week placement after finals during which time students shadow the PRHO whose job they will be taking.

Honours year   Intercalated degrees are offered at the end of the second year and occasionally after the third or fourth year. There is a wide range of bioscience subjects as well as healthcare ethics and law, history of medicine, and psychology. Students wishing to intercalate would be expected to have passed all exams at first sitting, and funding is allocated according to academic merit. Some scholarships are available from businesses depending on the subject studied.

Elective study/SSMs   In years 1 and 2 there is one two-week SSM per year. In year 3 and 4 there is one SSM per semester lasting 3 or 4 weeks. SSMs can be on practically anything, although in years 3 and 4 one must be in a DGH and one in the community. The Elective is in the final year and lasts 8 weeks. A project must be submitted upon returning to Manchester. Students are encouraged to go abroad.

Course organisation   Manchester was the first medical school in the UK to devote the curriculum to PBL. As a result the course is well established and efficiently run. However, in clinical years, organisation varies from hospital to hospital and firm to firm. Choice of placement is given, but first choice is not always guaranteed.

PRHO year   There are plenty of PRHO jobs in the Manchester area. There is a matching scheme and most people tend to stay in the region.

The learning environment

The university is 20 minutes walk from the city centre. Most accommodation is not more than 25 minutes walk from university, with most students choosing to live in Fallowfield, a student-orientated suburb. Base hospitals are all within 30 minutes of the university, and, though having a car is a definite advantage in clinical years, public transport is frequent and extensive.

Library facilities   The Medical Faculty Library is well equipped with the basic textbooks, but demand is high and it is often busy. It is open 9 a.m.–8 p.m. during term-time weekdays only. The John Rylands University Library across the road stocks most of the major journals. This library is open from 9 a.m.–9.30 p.m. weekdays, and 9 a.m. –6 p.m. and 1 p.m.–6 p.m. on Saturday and Sunday respectively. The opening hours in holiday times are shorter. Hospital libraries vary in size and standard.

Computer facilities   There are excellent computer facilities in the medical school and John Rylands Library, with internet access and email for all. A number of computer-assisted learning programs are available, and computer labs are open from 9 a.m.–7 p.m. Hospitals also have computer and email facilities.

Clinical skills laboratory   More and more emphasis is being placed on the use of skills labs, and facilities are being improved. There are a variety of mannequins for practising CPR, injections, blood taking, etc., and video resources on clinical skills.

Teaching hospitals   Student facilities vary between hospitals. There are normally eight students per firm, and staff are generally willing to teach, although an element of luck is involved here. Most hospitals used are in the Greater Manchester area.

Course details

Course length	5 years or 6 years pre-med
Total number of medical undergraduates	c. 1500
Male/Female ratio	n/a

Admission procedure

Average A level requirements	AAB
Average Scottish Higher requirements	AAAAB
Number of applicants (Sept 2000 entry)	1600
Proportion of applicants interviewed	60%
Make up of interview panel	3 consultants and 1 bioscientist or GP with a mix of specialities, gender and ethnicity
Months interviews held	Nov–April
Number admitted (Sept 2000 entry)	310
Proposed entry size for 2001	340
Proportion of overseas students	6%–7%
Proportion of mature students	10%
Faculty's view of taking a gap year	Neutral
Proportion taking Intercalated Hons	25–30 students each year
Possibility of direct entrance to clinical phase	Low

Finances

Tuition fees per year	£1050
Fees for self-funding students	£1050
Fees for graduates	£1050
Fees for overseas students	Pre-clinical–£9400 Clinical–£17 200
Assistance for elective funding	Scholarships and prizes available
Assistance for travel to attachments	Not via university
Access and hardship funds	Yes, via Dept. of Awards and Exams

Average cost of living

Weekly rent	Halls £45–£75 Private £35–£60
Pint of lager	Union Bar £1.40 City Centre pub £1.80
Cinema	£5 without student ID but all places give at least £1 off
Nightclub	Free–£20.00

Student friendliness and support   Faculty staff are very approachable and feedback is encouraged. Good relationships between students and tutors are fostered through tutorials. Student counselling services are available from the Union and they are highly regarded.

Student life

With a student population of 50 000, Manchester offers an endless choice of where to go and what to do. There is a wide variety of pubs, bars, clubs, stores, theatres and restaurants, each with a different character, theme or style. The city is multi-cultural and there is a good mix of home, overseas, mature and postgraduate students. There is also a vibrant gay and lesbian scene in Manchester. The music scene (post Acid and 'Madchester') is on the up and as well as the local scene, most of the big name tours include Manchester gigs. On the downside, living in a large city brings with it an increased risk of crime, and the university is situated between some high-risk areas.

Accommodation   University accommodation is guaranteed for first years, and, although most students choose to move into the private sector after this, many do stay. Halls may be catered or self-catering and vary in price and standard. There is a lot of private sector accommodation, ranging in price from £35 to £60 per week. Most accommodation is within walking distance of the university, and a short bus ride from the town centre.

Entertainment and societies   The Medical Students Representative Council (MSRC) is elected each year by students and organises a number of medics events throughout the year, including the famous pyjama pub crawl and the Annual Winter Ball. There are also year clubs which organise trips, parties, and one graduation ball for each year. The medics run an orchestra, a dramatic society, which organises an annual pantomime, and revue. *Mediscope* is the Manchester Medical School Magazine and it is now published on the web. This is published about three times a year. A huge range of clubs and societies are run from Manchester Students Union, which is very close to the faculty.

Sports facilities   Sport is popular in Manchester, especially football. Manchester City offers cut-priced tickets to students for home games and the majority of locals living in the student areas are City fans. There is also a discount price for students at Sales Sharks Rugby Club. Manchester's sports scene has benefited from the opening of many facilities built to cater for the Commonwealth Games. Developments include a velodrome and an Olympic swimming pool. There are medics rugby, hockey, tennis, netball and football teams. There is a strong emphasis on participation and socialising. The university has many sports clubs, but medics tend to play for the medics' team if one exists in their sport. A brilliant annual tour also takes place for each medics sport team.

City and surrounds   Because of the large student population in Manchester there are loads of student nights at clubs and pubs, and a number of student discounts are available in shops and restaurants. However, with the many benefits of city life come the pitfalls, which include the difficulty in getting away from it all. However, the Peak District, Pennines, Lake District and North Wales are not far away, nor are the competing cities of Liverpool, Leeds and Sheffield.

The five BEST things about Manchester Medical School

- Enthusiasm for medicine is maintained by a course which puts emphasis on clinical problems from day one.
- The Faculty staff are very approachable and open to change. There are plenty of opportunities to give feedback on both course and staff.
- The social life is excellent. There are loads of events organised by the MSRC and there is generally lots going on at reasonable prices.
- Manchester University is a multi-faculty institute, and its large site means that facilities are generally good.
- In the 3rd year a load of new people arrive from St Andrews, which spices things up a bit!

The five WORST things about Manchester Medical School

- Adjusting to self-directed learning can be difficult for some students who are used to being spoon fed.

- Some members of staff take the concept of self-directed learning too far, resulting in lack of teaching for students.

- Hospital placements are often quite a distance away and can be difficult to reach on public transport.

- Manchester does have a higher than average crime rate and insurance premiums are in the more expensive bands.

- There is anti-student sentiment felt by some of the locals.

Further information

Admissions: Admissions Officer
Faculty of Medicine
Stopford Building
University of Manchester
Oxford Road
Manchester
M13 9PT
General admissions Tel: 0161 275 2077
Fax: 0161 275 5697

Newcastle (Durham)

Newcastle is a friendly city and the University is very centrally situated. The medical school is 5 minutes away from the main campus, very near to the halls of residence. Like the rest of the university there is a wide range of students, national and international, from many different backgrounds. The staff are generally approachable and supportive and well liked by students. The course begins with integrated sciences and in the third year attachments apply this knowledge in a clinical context. Early patient contact comes from hospital and GP visits in the first two years. The social life, centred around both the university and the city itself, is excellent, with something to appeal to everyone. Newcastle, the northernmost English university city, gives a warm welcome to its students.

Changes to the course are planned with the introduction of the Stockton Campus in September 2001, and the medical school is currently undergoing building work at Newcastle. The building work is due to finish before the next intake.

Stop press

The universities of Newcastle and Durham are combining to run a new medical degree course which will integrate a new 2 year course at the Stockton campus of the University of Durham with the final three years (phase II) of the current medical degree course at Newcastle. The first students will begin at Durham in 2001.

Where possible we have given details for the Newcastle/Durham course:

Course length	• 5 years (2 years at Stockton campus and 3 years at Newcastle)
Total number of places	• 70 (2001 entry)
Admission requirements and process	• As for Newcastle
Weekly rent	• Halls £43.50 Private £28
Pint of lager	• Union £1.20 City Centre pub £1.50
Cinema	• £2.80 (with NUS card)
Nightclub	• 50p–£15

The course

In years 1 and 2 the course is systems based, becoming more clinically relevant as you progress through. There is no intention for the University to move towards solely problem-based learning, although the first two years of the course are set to include more case-based work, which will be added to and revisited in later years. The pre-clinical/clinical divide is reducing, and there are several opportunities for early patient contact in the form of project work, hospital and GP visits, and patient presentations. Practical skills, like taking blood, are taught from term 1 of the first year.

Clinical attachments on the wards begin at the start of the third year with the clinical skills course, followed by essential junior rotations, elective study and finally, essential senior rotations, covering all major clinical specialties.

Teaching and assessment   Currently In years 1 and 2 (phase 1) there are approximately 10 lectures each week, with small group seminar and practical sessions to support these. Anatomy classes use prosected specimens. Since the visit of the GMC in 1998, and the review of the curriculum that is underway, the intention is to decrease the timetabled hours in the first two years, leaving students more "white" time. Wednesday afternoons are free for sport. Examinations consist of a multiple choice exam, a data response paper and a "spotter" (OSCE). In phase 1, exams happen at the end of each semester, and about 6 weeks into the first year there is a short MCQ, which gives students a chance to see how they're doing. There are also several in-course assessments, and a Special Study Module is being introduced to phase 1. From 2001, 220 students will be based at the University of Newcastle, and 70 at University of Durham Stockton Campus for the first two years. Candidates should state on their UCAS form to which they are applying.

Phase 2: Third year sees the emphasis shift greatly to clinical experience. There is an introductory "Clinical Skills" course, lasting 16 weeks, which introduces students systematically and thoroughly to clinical history-taking and examination, and is one of the best received parts of the course by students. After "Clinical Skills" students embark on a series of Essential Junior Rotations, introducing them to the various clinical specialities. Fourth year begins with a block of teaching based at the medical school in Newcastle, before the Stage 3 exams. Candidates considering Newcastle should be aware that this structure for stage 3 will be new. Students will be attached to a "base unit" for the whole of 3rd year, and this will not necessarily be Newcastle, but one of four centres across the North. For students based far afield (for example on Teesside), this is likely to mean finding accommodation there for the year. Be wary of talking to current Newcastle students about third year – their experience will be very different. Stage 3 exams (early in year 4) consist of data/problem-solving papers, MCQ and an OSCE. In-course assessment is by way of marks for the Junior Rotations, and a 5000 word "Literature Review".

Stage 4 begins in January of the fourth year with 21 weeks of Student Selected Modules based in hospital, investigative and community medicine. SSMs are assessed by poster and oral presentation. The 9 week elective period (plus 2 weeks holidays) follows. Final year consists of Essential Senior Rotations in the major clinical specialties. Placements can be throughout the North – from Whitehaven in the West, to North Shields in the East, Bishop Auckland in the South, to Ashington in the North. Final year students spend five days a week in hospital and are expected to become part of the team to which they are attached, including being around during some evenings. The emphasis is on self-directed learning. Final exams at the end of fifth year consist of data interpretation, an OSCE and a "long case".

Placements outside the university   In years 1 and 2 all placements are local (Newcastle if on the Newcastle-based course, Teesside if in Stockton). In the clinical years attachments may be much further afield (see above) There is usually good accommodation provided. Travel expenses are currently partially reimbursed, although

Course details

Course length	5 years
Total number of undergraduates	965
Male/Female ratio	32 : 68 (1999 intake)

Admission procedure

Average A level requirements	AAB – must include Chemistry and/or Biology; the Medical School also requires at least AAAAB at GCSE, including Maths, Science and English Language
Average Scottish Higher requirements	AAAAB including English and Maths. The school also requires at least four at grade 1 and a grade 2 at standard grade, including Chemistry or Biology
Number of applicants (Sept 2000 entry)	1326
Proportion of applicants interviewed	c. 40%
Make-up of interview panel	Usually 2 academic staff (occasionally with 1 non-academic)
Months interviews held	Nov–March
Number admitted (Sept 2000 entry)	220
Proposed intake for 2001 (including Durham intake)	290
Proportion of overseas students	7%
Proportion of mature students	10–15%
Faculty's view of taking a gap year	Positive attitude (if used well)
Proportion taking Intercalated Hons	c. 7% (starting in 1999) normally higher
Possibility of direct entrance to clinical phase	Yes, but very competitive

Finances

Tuition fees per year	£1050
Fees for self-funding students	£1050 p.a.
Fees for graduates	£1050 p.a.
Fees for overseas students	£9190 p.a. (pre-clinical) and £17 015 p.a. (clinical)
Assistance for elective funding	No
Assistance for travel to attachments	Currently under review
Access and hardship funds	Some funds available via university registrar. (Some limited funds from medical school benefactors)

Average cost of living

Weekly rent	Halls £40–£60 self-catering Private £25–£60
Pint of lager	Union £1.30 City Centre pub £2
Cinema	£3.50 with union card
Nightclub	Free–£8

this is under review. Students may move elsewhere in the UK for special study modules in 4th year if they can provide evidence that the SSM would be unavailable in Newcastle.

Honours year   Students who do very well on the course are encouraged to intercalate, either after the second or fourth year, and study for the additional degree of BMedSci. Research projects are wide ranging, from clinical to lab-based work, and topics in the social sciences. There are currently 24 students who have taken this option.

Elective study/SSMs   An SSM is being introduced to phase 1. Stage 4 (year 4 term 2, after stage 3 exams) begins with three student-selected modules lasting 7 weeks each, where hospital, community and investigative based topics are studied in depth. This is followed by an 11 week elective period, usually spent abroad.

Course organisation   Handbooks (study-guides) are available for all four stages of the course which help students to know what specifically they need to learn. There are staff–student committees to discuss any changes to the curriculum and assessment process and students' voices do tend to be heard. Study guides are also available online, along with practice MCQ questions and other resources. Email-based mailing lists are the main way that the medical school communicates administrative issues to students. The ethos is very much based around letting someone know early if there is a problem – hence the personal tutor scheme and "Personal and Professional Development" strand of the course.

PRHO year   Students apply for house jobs at the end of the fourth year. There is some competition for the more popular posts, but there are more than enough jobs around the region. Most newly graduated doctors stay in or near to Newcastle for their house jobs. After graduation, there is a 2 week "PRHO shadowing course" to ease the transition from student to doctor, allow students to become familiar with the Trust in which they'll be working, and cover some practical aspects of being a PRHO.

The learning environment

The campus is situated very close to the city centre and includes the Royal Victoria Infirmary (adjoining the Medical School). There is ample opportunity to mix with non-medical students, whilst at the same time the facilities are good within the medical school (refectories, gym, etc).

Library facilities   The Medical Library is situated within the Medical School and is open until 10 p.m. during the week, but daytime only at weekends. It is well stocked with books and videos, but does get busy at exam time. Students may also use the University Library, which is also close to the Medical School (5 minutes walk).

Computer facilities   These tend to be very good, and much information is passed on to students via email. Computer courses are held as part of the course specifically in word processing and use of email/Internet searching databases. There are 120 general access PCs in the medical school with an additional eight stations for email only. Opening hours are the same as the library. If these are busy, there are numerous quieter clusters throughout the university available for use.

Clinical skills laboratory   Clinical skills are emphasised very early in the course and form an integral part of the exams. The lab is available for private revision sessions as well as timetabled teaching sessions.

Teaching hospitals   Ward groups of four to five students in the third year and one to three in years 4 and 5 are taught in hospitals around Newcastle and the North. Staff are generally keen to teach and welcome students, although reports are mixed.

Student friendliness and support   All students are assigned a personal tutor for pastoral support, and faculty staff are friendly and approachable. The University and Student's Union have a number of welfare officers and counselling services, including Nightline. All fresher medics join a peer family (often with five generations!) to help get themselves orientated.

Student life

Students at Newcastle quickly develop an affection for the city, and the large student presence in a small city makes for an excellent social life.

Accommodation   First year accommodation is guaranteed in halls or self-catering flats, although not all are centrally located. The housing office offers help and advice to students renting in the private sector, as most do from year 2. Popular student areas for renting are Jesmond, Heaton and Fenham.

Entertainment and societies   Medsoc events take place every Friday evening, and usually consist of a guest speaker or show followed by a free bar; karaoke nights, blind date, man-o-man. The annual Medsoc-Dentsoc challenge is a regular favourite. The third years stage a medics' revue in May, and there are numerous medics' balls and dinners throughout the year. A wide range of other societies are available through the Union.

Sports facilities   Medics rugby and hockey teams compete in leagues, and there are also netball, football, cricket, squash and other sports clubs for medics, and innumerable other university-run clubs. The medical school has its own gym, and the university sports facilities are good and close by. For the enthusiastic supporter, there is Newcastle United Football Club, as well as Rugby Union, basketball, and many more professional sports teams.

City and surrounds   Newcastle is a very lively but relatively small city located within easy reach of the hills of Northumberland and the north-east coast of England. Recently voted eighth best party town in the world, there is no shortage of bars and pubs, and an ever-increasing club scene. The Medical School has good access to the city centre shops, theatre, cinema, museums, art galleries and music venues. More shops are to be found at the Metrocentre just across the Tyne in Gateshead. The locals are generally very friendly and eager for everyone to have a good time. Crime does not seem to be a major problem in most areas, but bikes do get stolen from time to time.

The five BEST things about Newcastle Medical School

- Friendly locals in a small, but not tiny city, so the atmosphere is friendly and never impersonal.
- Cost of living is relatively low.
- If you need a break from city life, it's easy to escape to the country or the coast.
- New pubs, clubs and restaurants spring up all the time.
- Free beer at Medsoc.

The five WORST things about Newcastle Medical School

- There is anxiety about how the new developments with the Stockton Campus and the increase in student numbers might impact on course organisation and the student body.

- There is some local hostility to southerners (anyone from south of Sheffield).

- The exam system has been changed several times and this has had an unsettling effect – although the current system has been up and running for 3 years now.

- The tutor system doesn't work for everyone (efforts are being made to improve the scheme).

- Some consultants mutter bitterly words to the effect of "Of course, the students at Newcastle don't know any anatomy these days..." You'll get sick of hearing it.

Further information

Admissions: The Medical School
University of Newcastle
Framlington Place
Newcastle Upon Tyne
NE2 4HH
Course/admission enquiries Tel: 0191 222 7034
Fax: 0191 222 6139

950 students
Email: medschool@nottingham.ac.uk
www: http://www.nott.ac.uk

Nottingham

Nottingham is a campus university with a community atmosphere. Medics and non-medics mix in the first year in superb halls of residence on a beautiful campus. There is plentiful off-campus accommodation, which is well situated and very student orientated. The cost of living compares favourably with other university towns and the city is very vibrant and multicultural. The course is systems based with emphasis on the early introduction of clinical skills. Outside placements are accessible and the quality of teaching is high. All students do a BMedSci degree within the 5 year course and there are growing opportunities to study abroad. Clinical attachments are assessed individually and within themselves. The elective follows finals and this is a great idea. Most graduates have a job on the matching scheme and spend time shadowing initially.

The course

Nottingham has an integrated course with semesterly systems-based teaching for the first 2 years. One morning every fortnight is spent in general practice or in hospital, seeing patients with relevant problems and learning to take a history. Year 3 involves a research project leading to a BMedSci for everybody. A 1 week bridging course prepares students for the medical and surgical attachments that take up the rest of the third year, before the clinical speciality attachments of years 4 and 5. There is a large emphasis on personal and professional development comprising communication skills, ethics and careers.

Teaching and assessment   Large group lectures of variable quality are the basis of most first and second year courses. These are supplemented with a limited number of tutorials and seminars. Anatomy is taught by dissection and clinical problem solving. Practical classes are split and tele-linked. Exams are in January and June, and students are encouraged to give feedback that often results in improvements. Exams in the clinical years follow each attachment and work done during the attachment is recorded in logbooks. There is no 1st and 2nd MB as such, and finals consist only of medicine, surgery and clinical laboratory sciences. Continual assessment has obvious benefits, but their use does mean that exams and their associated stresses happen often.

Placements outside the university   There are some visits in years 1 and 2, which require travelling, and students are helped with the organisation. Clinical attachments are mostly in Nottinghamshire, at University Hospital, City Hospital (5 miles) and Mansfield (20 miles), but Derby (15 miles) and Lincoln (30 miles) are also used. Students often share cars and there are very few problems with transport.

Honours year   There is no Honours year option as everyone at Nottingham does a BMedSci (Hons) degree with the research component in year 3. This can give individuals an option to leave medicine with a qualification after this. This option is rarely taken. Some students present their projects at conferences and a few publish papers on their work. Most students enjoy their research projects, a few tolerate them and a small number can't wait for them to be over.

Nottingham

Course details

Course length	● 5 years
Total number of medical undergraduates	● 966
Male/Female ratio	● 35:65

Admission procedure

Average A level requirements	● AAB (Chemistry and Biology at A Grade plus one other mainstream A level)
Average Scottish Higher requirements	● AAABB including Biology, Chemistry and Physics at this level, CSYSs equate with A level requirements
Number of applicants (Sept 2000 entry)	● 3450
Proportion of applicants interviewed	● 20%
Make up of interview panel	● 2 assessors (GPs, clinicians, academics)
Months interviews held	● Nov–March
Number admitted (Sept 2000 entry)	● 212
Proposed entry size for 2001	● 228
Proportion of overseas students	● 10–15%
Proportion of mature students	● 10–15%
Faculty's view of taking a gap year	● Encouraged, due to length of training and experience which can be gained
Proportion taking Intercalated Hons	● All students do a BMedSci degree
Possibility of direct entrance to clinical phase	● No

Finances

Tuition fees per year	● £1050
Fees for self-funding students	● £1050 p.a.
Fees for graduates	● £1050 p.a.
Fees for overseas students	● £9400 p.a. (pre-clinical) and £17230 (clinical)
Assistance for elective funding	● Some in exceptional circumstances
Assistance for travel to attachments	● None from University
Access and hardship funds	● Yes

Average cost of living

Weekly rent	● Halls £40–£93 Private £40–£70
Pint of lager	● Union Bar £1.40 City Centre pub £2.20
Cinema	● £3–5
Nightclub	● £1–£5 weekdays (posh clubs charge more at the weekend)

Elective study/SSMs   The elective is at the end of all attachments and exams in year 5. Most people choose a mixture of work and play, and a brief report is expected from everyone. There are two SSMs of 5 weeks in the 5th year, choice is good and there are options to study in Europe.

Course organisation   The current course at Nottingham has been established since the early 1990s and the organisation is reasonably good. Faculty is very receptive to suggestions and criticism of the course.

PRHO year   The computer-matching scheme finds a job for the majority of graduates. Most posts are local, and additional, more distant, posts are being increased in number, with jobs in Truro, Taunton, the Isle of Man and Hull. The scheme is currently under review.

The learning environment

The Medical School is part of a large vibrant and modern university. The School is located in a wing of the Queen's Medical Centre (University Hospital), one of the largest teaching hospitals in Europe. It is linked by a footbridge to the university campus and is within walking distance of hall accommodation, sports facilities and the Union. On the other side of the hospital is the main student residential area, Lenton. Bus links to the city centre and other hospitals are good. The Medical School, being part of a hospital, has a fairly clinical feel; the climate is subtropical and there is no bar.

Library facilities   The library is large, carpeted, but lacking daylight. It is open until 11.15 p.m. and during the day at weekends. It is well stocked with core texts and journals but becomes very busy at exam time, when overflow facilities come into use.

Computer facilities   IT facilities are excellent, with over 200 terminals. There is free access to the internet, CD-Roms, and computer-assisted learning packages for teaching and revision. The IT lab is open 24 hours. Facilities are improving at outlying hospitals.

Clinical skills laboratory   The lab is staffed and resources have grown rapidly. It is used on a casual basis and has many self-teaching aids – models of eyes, ears, arms (for blood pressure) and breasts, etc.

Teaching hospitals   The facilities, such as student common rooms, canteen food and the accommodation, are generally better in the peripheral hospitals than at the larger teaching centres. It is generally felt that the standard of teaching and the friendliness of staff are better away from the teaching hospital.

Student friendliness and support   Pastoral care is taken very seriously, with tutor and mentoring systems involving both staff and senior students. Whether or not you see your tutor and mentor can, in some cases, be "a bit hit and miss" and this sometimes undermines the system. Faculty office is usually open, but often vacant(!). The university and Students Union have welfare and counselling services, and some legal help is available from Union solicitors.

Student life

The main distinguishing feature of medics' life at Nottingham is the extent to which medical students are interspersed within the whole university population. Many medics live with their friends from hall after the first year. Lenton, the main student area, is well equipped with cheapish pubs, laundrettes, 24-hour shops, take-aways and buses. Although the campus accommodation is excellent, the university could take more responsibility for housing off-campus. Student life is rich and varied, and there is plenty of time to enjoy it whilst doing a medical degree. The MedSoc provides a good range of social events, balls and guest lectures.

Accommodation   Almost all first years are housed in university accommodation (single rooms with telephones) in catered halls or self-catering flats. There are 12 medium sized halls, each with their own bar, giving campus a semi-collegiate yet integrated feel. In subsequent years you can apply to stay in halls or have the option of flats. Most second years live in private rented houses; 80% live in the same, relatively safe area, 20 minutes walk from campus and town. House-hunting begins after Christmas, and, despite the university housing scheme, most students organise it themselves without university vetting. The Union organises house-hunting for first years wanting to live out.

Entertainment and societies   There are hundreds of university clubs and societies facilitating much interaction within the student body, notably Cocksoc (cocktails not animal husbandry!). Nottingham has the largest student rag in the country called *Karni*. On-campus entertainment revolves around hall life and includes bars and themed parties. In later years, the pub and club scenes dominate. MedSoc organises parties, which facilitate inter-year mixing, and guest lectures.

Sports facilities   There are good quality, accessible facilities at Nottingham. Medics teams are particularly strong in hockey, rugby, tennis and football, and most sports are represented somewhere in the university. All standards are catered for, and clubs provide a focus for excellent social lives.

City and surrounds   The city centre is compact, with good shopping. Nottingham is renowned for its inexpensive and diverse bars, clubs, pubs and restaurants. The theatres are good, but there are few live music venues. The city centre is within walking distance of most off-campus accommodation, and a 10-minute bus ride from campus. The city is relatively safe and student friendly. It is central, and rail links to the rest of the Midlands and London are good. The Peak District, and countryside that borders Nottingham, provides a welcome escape where students can risk life and limb far away from biochemistry revision.

The five BEST things about Nottingham Medical School

- Established integrated course which evolves through with feedback from the students.
- Good social life for students, with variety, value and accessibility.
- Beautiful campus, with good community spirit and healthy inter-hall rivalry.
- Integration of medics with non-medics in halls broadens social circles and reduces the cliquiness that medics are sometimes accused of!
- Lack of a Medical School bar leads to a better mixed social life outside of medicine.

The five WORST things about Nottingham Medical School

- Due to the poor union bar with no venue for top bands there is little to attract medics back to campus after their first year!
- It is widely felt that the university attracts students of a similar background, leading to a lack of diversity within the student population.
- Lack of student facilities in the main teaching hospitals, such as common rooms, cheap food and quality accommodation, compared to some of the luxury elsewhere.

- Low levels of feedback and poor course co-ordination undermines a systematic approach to assessment – especially with regards to the third year project.

- The pre-clinical course is too lecture based, with not enough seminars and tutorials.

Further information

Admissions: Admissions Officer
Medical and Health Sciences Faculty Office
University Park
University of Nottingham
Nottingham
NG7 2RD
Tel: 0115 970 9379 Fax: 0115 970 9922
Online prospectus http://www.nottingham.ac.uk/mhs-faculty-office

Nottingham

Oxford

Oxford is a unique place. If you would like to live in either modern accomodation or in 15th century halls and meet students of all backgrounds; have the double benefits of a small College and a large University; and want to study a traditional, yet innovative, medical course, then Oxford is for you!

Some may criticise the lack of clinical involvement during the first 3 years of study here. However, the firm scientific basis of medicine is of vital importance and the acquisition of skills, such as the critical evaluation of papers and an understanding of research, are all rightly given very high priority. Three years before significant patient contact may seem like a long time to some, but the knowledge and skills gained during the pre-clinical course will be of use for the rest of your career.

The course demands the very highest level of academic ability and commitment. However, your college tutor, who selects you in the first place, has a vested interest in your success and, in most cases, works very hard on your behalf – no one is left to struggle. The short terms and long holidays also make the hard work survivable and enjoyable.

The course

Oxford Medical School was recently assessed by the QAA as a single 6 year course, but for practical purposes, there remains a clear-cut division between the pre-clinical and clinical courses in Oxford. At present in the pre-clinical school, the first five terms are spent studying the basic medical sciences (anatomy, biochemistry, physiology, pathology and neuroscience), and the final four terms working for an honours degree. (The timetable for the first 2 years is currently under review but the subjects will remain the same.) Application to the clinical school is competitive with about 55–65% of the Oxford pre-clinical students staying on. The rest go mainly to London or Cambridge, and there is an influx of students from elsewhere, mainly Cambridge, with additions from London and the Scottish medical schools.

The clinical course lasts 3 years and aims to deliver the best teaching of both scientific principles and clinical practice. It is in a particularly good position to do so, because of the combination of its small size and the very high quality of its academic and clinical staff. Year 4 consists of a medicine, surgery, and an 8 week laboratory medicine course (pathology), together with a residential general practice attachment, ethics and communication skills. Special Study Modules are an exciting and innovative addition to the fourth year; they are in such diverse subjects as Philosophy, Theology, Chronic Illness and Creativity, where students are free to explore their interests.

Year 5 contains all the specialist rotations, such as paediatrics and psychiatry. Year 6 focuses again on medicine and surgery, with a 10 week elective period, 14 weeks of Clinical Special Study Modules and a 6 week PRHO shadowing at a DGH.

There is a great deal of ward-based teaching, both with consultants and the more junior doctors (all of whom are keen to practice being teaching hospital consultants!). The modular form of the specialist rotations means that there is no easy fifth year, but the pressure at finals is much reduced. At present, as almost all the clinical students are in Oxford at any one time, there is a strong sense of group identity and a very full social life. If the plans to expand the clinical school are put into full effect, it is not clear what impact this may have on this aspect of "the Oxford experience".

Teaching and assessment   In the pre-clinical years the basic medical sciences are taught by lectures and practicals, supported by most colleges giving tutorials with two to three students, two to three times a week. Currently, the assessments are at the end of the first year and before Easter in the 2nd year, and consist of essay papers, short notes and problem-solving questions. The practicals are assessed continuously and practical books must be kept up to date.

The third year course is taught in a similar way to the pre-clinical course, but allows much more time for personal study and the freedom to follow your academic interests. During this time, most students complete a research project, which often leads to publication in scientific journals. The course is assessed at the end of the third year (more essay papers), and students receive a classified BA(Hons).

At clinical level, the emphasis is much more on small group teaching and continuous assessment. The laboratory medicine course is taught by lectures and practicals, and is, on the whole, well taught and enjoyed. In the fifth year the specialties are assessed individually at the end of each placement, usually by clinical and written papers. So, in finals (at the end of the sixth year), some of these subjects are not reassessed. This significantly reduces the pressure at finals and few students fail.

Honours year   All students spend the last terms of the pre-clinical phase working for an honours degree in physiology or psychology (unless they are already graduates). The degree course has a large amount of flexibility, and students are encouraged to follow courses that interest them.

Placements outside Oxford   Except for the PRHO shadowing at the DGHs in the sixth year, the whole course can be taken in Oxford. Many find this very useful as it allows them to be involved in university and college life, whether sports, drama, music or other activities. There are, however, ample opportunities to travel (in addition to the elective) for those who want to: for example, several of the specialties (such as paediatrics and deliveries in obstetrics) can be studied in other parts of the country or world.

Elective study/SSMs   There is a 10 week elective in the sixth year and most go abroad. Some of the colleges can help financially. The 14 weeks of SSMs in final year are more clinical in nature than the modules of the first clinical year. There are over 60 options ranging from the traditional (e.g. cardiology, anaesthetics, general practice) to the innovative (creativity in healthcare, medical publishing, medical anthropology or even a language), and can be either purely clinical, research or a mixture of both. Even if the extensive list does not cover the one subject that you desperately want to study, you are free, with the Medical School's permission, to arrange your own.

Course details

Course length	● 6 years
Total number of undergraduates	● 600
Male/Female ratio	● 45:55

Admission procedure

Average A Level requirements	● AAA (including Chemistry)
Average Scottish Higher requirements	● 5 A grades and CSYS or A level passes (including Chemistry)
Number of applicants (Sept 1999 entry)	● Pre-clinical 600 Clinical 138
Proportion of applicants interviewed	● Pre-clinical 80% Clinical 100%
Make-up of interview panel	● Pre-clinical: 1 or 2 College Fellows (may be several interviews) Clinical: panel of 4 including clinicians, a pre-clinical teacher, and at least one woman
Months interviews held	● Pre-clinical: Dec Clinical: late Jan/early Feb
Numbers admitted (Sept 1999 entry)	● Pre-clinical 113 Clinical 104
Proposed entry for 2002	● Pre-clinical 150
Proportion of overseas students	● 7% (quota)
Proportion of mature students	● 4–6% (no quota)
Faculty's view of taking a gap year	● Generally supportive if for good reasons, but consult individual college admission tutors
Proportion taking Intercalated Hons	● 100%. The Honours degree is an integral part of the course
Possibility of direct entrance to clinical phase	● Yes (Honours graduates only with pre-clinical qualifications)

Finances

Tuition fees per year	● University fee £1050 (means tested) EU students £1050 Non-EU students also pay college fees, about £1500 (clinical) and £3500 (pre-clinical) – varies between Colleges
Fees for self-funding students	● £1050 p.a.
Fees for overseas students	● £9133 p.a. (pre-clinical) £16 745 p.a. (clinical)
Assistance for elective funding	● Very helpful financially and otherwise. Colleges also have funds
Assistance for travel between attachments	● Yes
Access and hardship funds	● Available, especially if unforeseen circumstances cause hardship

Average cost of living

Weekly rent	● Halls vary, but normally less than the private sector Private £60
Pint of lager	● Union £1–£1.50 City Centre pub £1.80–£2.50
Cinema	● £3.50–£4.50
Nightclub	● Free–£7

Course organisation   The clinical school is well organised; the "powers that be" are very friendly, approachable and more than open to suggestions on how to improve the course. This is, in general, how the clinical course has developed.

PRHO Year   House officer jobs in Oxford hospitals are allocated by a computerised matching scheme in which the majority of students get one job in Oxford. The scheme is operated early enough for students to then apply to other areas where there are larger numbers of PRHO jobs. The matching scheme is only open to Oxford medical students.

The learning environment

Oxford University takes great pains in its selection process, and you will meet a wide range of students from all over the country and from many walks of life. The early years are spent studying basic medical sciences in and around the centre of Oxford. This is amidst the Oxford colleges with their long traditions of study and learning. The clinical school is based at the John Radcliffe Hospital (JR), which is a large teaching hospital situated in Headington, 2 miles east of Oxford city centre. The JR is one of the country's finest hospitals, and a very pleasant place to work, as it was designed with modern clinical practice in mind.

Fast Track Medicine for Bioscience Graduate Students

Oxford is starting a fast-track medical course for graduates from 2001. In the first year, it is expected that 10 students will be admitted, thereafter rising to 20 students annually. The course is only open to honours graduates in biosciences (a list of acceptable undergraduate degrees is in the prospectus); however, honours graduates of all disciplines may apply to the traditional course, completing it in 5 rather than 6 years by missing out the honours year in that course. Bioscience graduates may apply to both the fast-track and the traditional course if they wish.

The first year of the course will be spent studying basic medical sciences. This will be taught at the John Radcliffe site. Students will then join the clinical phase during years two to four. College tutorials will supplement the first year course and provision will be made for students to integrate efficiently into the clinical years.

Applications are to be made via UCAS; this year there were 150 applicants and 45 were interviewed for the 10 places.

During the first year, students will be liable to pay both the University fee (c. £1050) and the College fee (c. £3500); during the final three years only the University fee is payable and means-tested NHS bursaries are available. Foreign students will be required to pay the pre-clinical University fee (c. £9133) and College fee in the first year, and then only the clinical University fee (c. £16 745) annually during the latter part of the course. Students will be full members of an Oxford college throughout the course.

Further information may be obtained from the Medical School website, or the University Offices.

Library facilities   Oxford is very well catered for with respect to libraries, being a legal deposit. At pre-clinical level, the Radcliffe Science Library (RSL) and college libraries are the most useful and used. College facilities vary but are in general good to excellent. The RSL has an incredible number of books and journals, but rather limited opening hours out of term. The Cairns Library is located at the JR, and is the library used during clinical years. It is very well stocked and is open 24 hours a day, 365 days a year.

Computing facilities   The computing facilities are very good in colleges, departments, libraries and, at clinical level, in Osler House and the Cairns Library, where a large number of computers are reserved exclusively for medical students. Computer-assisted learning is soon to be introduced.

Clinical skills laboratory   This has just been introduced at the clinical school and has proved useful.

Teaching hospitals   The hospitals used are the John Radcliffe Hospital, which is modern and large; the Churchill Hospital and the Radcliffe Infirmary, which are older hospitals, The Nuffield Orthopaedic Hospital, The Warneford and Littlemore psychiatric hospitals.

Student friendliness and support   The university tutoring system works well in the pre-clinical years because of the collegiate system. In clinical years, when links with the college are not as strong, the system does not work so well but is supplemented by the excellent support, be it academic or pastoral, from the Medical School. Colleges provide significant financial assistance, ranging from subsidised accommodation, meals and entertainment, to elective funding and hardship grants. Oxford University has welfare and counselling facilities in addition to the provision by the Medical School and colleges.

Student life

At both pre-clinical and clinical levels, the small year size (about 100) means that medical students tend to know each other very well. Depending on your view point, this can either be an advantage or disadvantage, but most seem to enjoy the camaraderie and banter, whether in the bar or the dissection room! One of the great things about Oxford is the collegiate system: this broadens your horizons and makes it very easy to make friends with non-medics. At the clinical level, Osler House provides a very relaxed way of meeting people and making friends.

Accommodation   Pre-clinical students will find their life completely integrated with that of students in other subjects and will live with them in college accommodation. Many of the college buildings are old and beautiful, though do bear in mind that sometimes the accommodation you will actually live in will either be 1950s or private lodgings. All the accommodation is of a reasonable to good or excellent standard and fairly cheap.

Things are very different for clinical students however. Very few live on college sites as the majority of graduate accommodation is off site in nearby annexes. The exception is Green College, which was established for medical students and is still largely populated by them. (About a third of the clinical students live in Green College accommodation.) Many prefer to live out during their clinical training as it affords more independence than college can provide and there is plenty of good quality private accommodation in Oxford.

Entertainment and societies   There are numerous university and college based clubs and societies dedicated to ensuring that students get the most they can out of their time in Oxford. At pre-clinical these often form a prominent part of most people's social life with the medical society (MedSoc) supplementing this. The societies range from the sublime to the ridiculous, and you will find talents that catered for you never realised you had.

The clinical school social life tends to revolve around Osler House – a 1920s house in the grounds of the John Radcliffe run for and by clinical students. There is a bar, a television room, computing facilities, pool table and a pleasant garden. The Osler Committee organises many events – social, sporting and cultural. Many clinical students remain involved in other aspects of university life, and the fact that there is very little obligation to leave Oxford for long periods makes this much easier than at some other clinical schools. The clinical school pantomime, *Tingewick*, deserves a special mention. This occurs every year and is a great chance for the students to get their own back at their consultants and anyone else who deserves parody.

Sports facilities   Oxford is famous for its rowing and rugby, but other sports are well represented too. In particular, the collegiate structure means that there are both facilities and opportunities for involvement in sport at any level of ability. All the colleges have sports pitches and boat houses, and many can provide squash and tennis courts as well. Inter-collegiate competitions (Cuppers) form one focus for the competitive energy and the very committed will find themselves competing at the highest levels – the Varsity competitions. Even if you lack speed, strength, skill, accuracy or talent in general, you will still be able to find a team of your level and skill! In the collegiate events, the clinical school is represented by the Osler-Green teams who regularly manage to field competitive sides.

City and surrounds   Oxford, the city of "dreaming spires" is a small city with easy access to the rest of the country, and London in particular (coach only takes 90 minutes). Many pre-clinical students survive the first 3 years without needing to travel more than 5 minutes from the centre of the city, but at clinical school you are forced to move a little further afield. The town centre has the usual core of shops, and you will find it sufficient for most needs. Having said that, it doesn't compare to most "real" cities for variety. Culturally there is a lot going on, particularly if you like theatre and music. It has to be said that the club scene in Oxford is not very exciting and wouldn't suit the more dedicated punter, but you can get to and from London on buses leaving every 12 minutes, 24 hours a day.

The five BEST things about Oxford Medical School

- The Collegiate system – meeting students in a variety of subjects which predisposes to broader interests and education.

- Tutorial system: having 1 to 1 or 2 to 1 tuition, with the academic support that offers. Consequently, very few students fall behind in their work.

- Most of the teaching is in Oxford – this has a sociability value (you will see all of your friends all of the time) and helps with keeping travel costs down.

- Excellent scientific and clinical teaching together with a stimulating environment in a university with a first-class, worldwide reputation.

- Oxford is a beautiful city in which to work and, together with its traditions, make Oxford a unique and rare experience.

The five WORST things about Oxford Medical School

- The tourists!

- The public perception of Oxford is innacurate and unhelpful – don't be discouraged from applying!

- Some students at Oxford are incredibly hard working, so the pressure can build up at times.

- The nightlife in Oxford is a little limited.

- The scientific nature of the course, particularly during the preclinical years, does not suit everyone.

Further Information

Admissions Pre-clinical: The University Offices
Wellington Square
Oxford
OX1 2JD
Oxford Colleges Admission Service Tel: 01865 270207
Fax: 01865 270208
http://www.ox.ac.uk

Clinical Medical School Offices
John Radcliffe Hospital
Headington
Oxford
OX3 9DU
http://www.jr2.ox.ac.uk/medsch/

365 students
Email: admissions@st-and.ac.uk
www: http://www.st-and.ac.uk

St Andrews

Established in the 15th Century, St Andrews is the oldest university in Scotland. It is set in a small picturesque town on the east coast of Fife. The course lasts for 3 years, during which the importance of the traditional pre-clinical subjects is emphasised. After this the vast majority of students head south for Manchester where they complete their clinical studies (a further 3 years). The uniqueness of such a course provides a great opportunity for students to experience studying both in an ancient university town and a big vibrant city. The faculty is small and students socialise with medics and non-medics alike.

The course

St Andrews is the oldest university in Scotland, which explains the traditions and customs that surround being a student here. The course is quite traditional, being departmentalised rather than integrated but it is frequently reviewed and improved to suit the needs of a modern doctor in training. The first two years are spent learning anatomy and physiology. Cellular and Molecular Biology has recently been introduced to replace biochemistry. Second year students also choose a SSM in the second semester which is usually in the form of a project. The third year is spent studying Microbiology, Pharmacology, Public Health, and Applied Medical Science. Behavioural Sciences has been introduced in 2000 to replace Psychology and this course runs through the 3 years. You graduate in medical sciences, and then choose your clinical school for a further 3 years before graduating as a doctor. There is a guaranteed place at Manchester and the vast majority go there, but you are quite at liberty to apply to another school for your clinical studies.

Teaching and assessment   Teaching is by lectures, tutorials and practicals, with some tutorials using computer-based teaching. Anatomy is taught using cadavers, which the students dissect. Exams are varied and often include a mixture of MCQs, short-answer questions, essays, case studies and vivas. In years 1 and 2 exemptions can be gained, in which a score of more than 60% lets you off being tested on semester 1 material again in May.

Placements outside the university   Students are attached to a local GP clinic in the second year, and there are also two hospital visits as part of the course in the third year.

Honours year   An intercalated year is possible at the end of the third year for those who wish to convert their BSc into an Honours degree. Approximately 10% stay on for this additional year, including most of those who wish to apply to medical schools other than Manchester for their clinical studies.

St Andrews

Elective study/SSMs   The electives are taken at the clinical school you attend. Special Study Modules in medicine are being introduced to the course. Opportunities for studying modules in subjects such as Philosophy, Ethics, Pastoral Care and Counselling do exist, as well as more scientific areas (for example Histology).

Course details

Course length	● 3 years (clinical component completed elsewhere)
Total number of medical undergraduates	● 365
Male/Female ratio	● 50:50

Admission procedure

Average A level requirements	● ABB
Average Scottish Higher requirements	● AAABB
Number of applicants (Sept 2000 entry)	● 572
Proportion of applicants interviewed	● Only graduate, mature and Access applicants are normally interviewed
Make up of interview panel	● 3–4 Staff; admissions tutor, clinicians and lecturers (including a representative of an ethnic minority)
Months interviews held	● December–March
Number admitted (Sept 2000 entry)	● 112
Proposed entry size for 2001	● 120
Proportion of overseas students	● 8.5%
Proportion of mature students	● 10%
Faculty's view of taking a gap year	● Time should be used constructively, although not necessarily in healthcare related environment. Travel is encouraged
Proportion taking Intercalated Hons	● 10%
Possibility of direct entrance to clinical phase	● No clinical school at St Andrews

Finances

Tuition fees per year	● £1050
Fees for self-funding students	● £1050
Fees for graduates	● £2740
Fees for overseas students	● £11 950
Assistance for elective funding	● No elective during course at St Andrews
Assistance for travel to attachments	● (see profile)
Access and hardship funds	● Some support available (e.g. small interest free loans)

Average cost of living

Weekly rent	● Halls £38–£80 Private £50–£55
Pint of lager	● Union Bar £1.60 City Centre pub £2
Cinema	● £3
Nightclub	● Union nightclub (*megabop*) £2

Course organisation   The course still has a very traditional pre-clinical feel. There is little patient contact, although clinical relevance is always emphasised. The small class size for tutorials and dissection gives a great opportunity to develop good relationships between students and with staff. Some aspects of the course mimic the problem-based learning approach in operation at Manchester, and integration between the two schools has improved greatly over the last few years. One of the benefits of the course structure at St Andrew's is that students leave here with a degree whether or not they continue medical studies.

PRHO year   St Andrews students have the luxury of not needing to worry about house officer jobs. You may have some idea about where you would like to work, and you should consider this when you move on to the clinical school.

The learning environment

The Medical School consists of buildings scattered all around the town. They are all within walking distance of each other, so there is no problem getting around.

Library facilities   Opening hours are: Monday to Thursday 9 a.m.–10 p.m., Friday to Saturday 9 a.m.–6 p.m; and Sunday 1 p.m.–7 p.m. A reasonable range of texts is available, but many students buy the core texts due to the restricted availability of some titles.

Clinical skills laboratory   Access is good and the staff are helpful, although some of the facilities are a little dated.

Computer facilities   There are several computer rooms available and halls of residence have computer facilities. The university runs a 24 hour service.

Teaching hospitals   See Manchester or other universities that allow entry for the clinical phase.

Student friendliness and support   This is an area of major strength at St Andrews. In such a small town the medics are well integrated into the university, and you will have the chance to get to know everyone at the school and make friends outside the Faculty. The Dean and Faculty are good and very supportive (if perhaps a little inflexible), and tend to get to know everyone by name quite quickly. The Students Union provides welfare and counselling services, including a "Nightline" service for stressed students. The locals tend to be student friendly, if only because the university is the biggest local employer and we almost outnumber the locals. However, when the revelry surrounding some of the ancient traditions still upheld by the university gets a bit over the top, town and gown relations can become a little strained.

Student life

St Andrews is a beautiful coastal town, with a population of less than 20 000, and is famed for its golf. Being the oldest of Scotland's four ancient universities, it has more than its share of traditions, and some of the oldest student societies. The students all live very near the centre of town, so it is never far to walk to meet a friend. There is a very good atmosphere amongst the students, with plenty of chances to mix with medics and non-medics, and enough things going on in the town, at the Union and with the societies, to keep you as busy as you want to be. Tourists and golf followers can make the town bustle a bit too much at times, but you can go celebrity spotting with some success.

Accommodation   All students can spend their first year in university accommodation (halls and flats), and there are often rooms available for further years. Rooms are often shared and the standard of flats is generally good. Some halls are better than others, but none are bad. Other privately owned accommodation is available, for which the university has no control, and rents average at £50–55 a week. Parking is difficult if you want to live in the town centre. There is a housing office at the university which can help you find places.

Entertainment and societies   The Union is okay – especially for freshers getting to know the place – and alcohol is very cheap, but the club scene is lacking, with very few bands or comedians. Occasionally, the Union will arrange some visiting top DJs (such as Cream regulars). Medsoc (called "The Bute") has good socials, including a famed Ball as well as a raucous revue. There are lots of different types of societies, from the very sensible to the downright silly. Social life tends to focus around balls and events run by these societies. There is normally something each and every week.

Sports facilities   Most sports are supported, especially hockey and rugby, and there is a medics competition every year, called the "Hypertrophy". Medical school teams do not play every week, and keen players often get involved with their hall teams or the main university clubs. Inter-hall competitions are also popular. The facilities have been improved in recent years, such as the gym and athletics union. There is no university swimming pool. It is, of course, golf heaven, with the Royal and Ancient offering excellent deals for students. Entrance to many top-class competitions is free to students wearing the traditional red gowns.

City and surrounds   The town has easily enough pubs, restaurants and cafes to keep most people happy, but ravers and shopaholics will have to travel to Edinburgh or Dundee for some real action. Outdoor types have easy access to the Grampians, and the nearby sea and beaches can be good fun. There is no railway station at St Andrews.

The five BEST things about St Andrews Medical School

- Beautiful town with a great atmosphere and easy access to the rest of Scotland.

- Medics have the opportunity to mix with other students.

- You get to see different types of university life, due to the move to another medical school for the clinical phase.

- The Bute Medical Society – our Medsoc – is excellent.

- Golf – if you happen to like golf.

The five WORST things about St Andrews Medical School

- Limited patient contact and low clinical content to course work.

- No night clubs, if you discount the Union.

- Not many shops – you will probably shop in your home town or travel to Dundee.

- It can get a bit cold at times.

- Golf – if you happen not to like golf – and the associated tourists.

Further information

Admissions: Admissions Office
79 North Street
St Andrews
Fife
KY15 9AJ
Schools Liaison Service Tel: 01334 462 150
University Admissions Tel: 01334 476 161
Fax: 01334 463 395

1000 students
Email: rs@sheffield.ac.uk
www: http: //www.sheffield.ac.uk

Sheffield

Sheffield, a city built on seven hills – like Rome – and almost as scenic! Sheffield University has a very large undergraduate population (15 000+) and is, reputedly, one of the best student cities in Britain (see *The Virgin Alternative Guide to British Universities*) and that's including the big place down south. The majority of students live and work in the scenic, i.e. hilly, parts of town, but there are a wide variety of areas to choose from. The Medical School attracts students from all walks of life and there is a good mixture of backgrounds represented. It uses a systems-based teaching scheme, running since 1994, which is under regular review. In general the curriculum can be looked upon as being a hybrid of the traditional science-based course and the newer problem-based approach, with increasing emphasis on self-directed learning. There tends to be one set of exams at the end of each year, and some project work is undertaken in groups throughout the course of the year.

The course

The course is divided into "pre-clinical" (years 1 and 2) and clinical (years 3-5) phases. A Foundation (i.e. pre-medical) year is also available for non-science students, confusingly referred to as either year 0 or year 1. The pre-clinical course is split into distinct 6-week modules which concentrate on a body system and contain teaching from anatomy, biochemistry, physiology and pharmacology, etc. Some ward visits have now been introduced.

The clinical course has been redesigned to increase the number of ward attachments but decrease the time spent on each attachment. Again, teaching is systems based and the traditional medicine/surgery divide has been abolished. These changes have given students a broader range of experience and teaching, but have reduced the opportunity to settle into a placement.

Teaching and assessment   The emphasis at Sheffield is on teaching broad concepts rather than detailed facts. This relies on the students' desire to look things up for themselves and hopefully produces doctors who genuinely enjoy their subject. There is a lot of anatomy dissection, with plenty of opportunity to get `hands on` experience, as well as practicals in physiology and biochemistry. Animals are not used in the lab, although animal products are. The number of lectures has been decreased to allow time for small group project work and self-directed learning. Clinical years consist mostly of ward-based attachments, interspersed with lecture blocks and tutorials.

Assessment of pre-clinical students is mainly by the end of year exams, which comprise written multiple choice papers and practical spotter exams to test anatomy, but there is also some continuous assessment through projects and practical write-ups. There are also brief anonymous tests at the end of each module, which are used as a means to monitor your own progress. In the clinical years, Objective Structure Clinical Exams (OSCEs) are added as well as written papers, and used to examine clinical skills.

Placements outside the university   Throughout the clinical phase there are peripheral attachments in hospitals throughout South Yorkshire and Humberside (up to 50 miles away). There is also an 8-week attachment with

---

Course details

Course length	● 5 years
Total number of medical undergraduates	● 1000
Male/Female ratio	● 43:57

Admission procedure

Average A level requirements	● ABB (A in Chemistry + B in another science subject)
Average Scottish Higher requirements	● AAAAB + CSYS (A in Chemistry and B in at least one other science)
Number of applicants (Sept 2000 entry)	● 2500 (for both A104 and A106 courses)
Proportion of applicants interviewed	● 32%
Make up of interview panel	● Medically qualified member of staff, biomedical scientist, medical student
Months interviews held	● Mid November to mid March
Number admitted (Sept 2000 entry)	● 223
Proposed entry size for 2001	● 238
Proportion of overseas students	● 7%
Proportion of mature students	● n/a
Faculty's view of taking a gap year	● Applicants not disadvantaged if gap year taken
Proportion taking Intercalated Hons	● 1.6%
Possibility of direct entrance to clinical phase	● Yes, if places available

Finances

Tuition fees per year	● £1050
Fees for self-funding students	● £1050
Fees for graduates	● £1050
Fees for overseas students	● £9300 p.a. (pre-clinical) £17 000 p.a. (clinical)
Assistance for elective funding	● Yes, bursaries and loans available
Assistance for travel to attachments	● No
Access and hardship funds	● Yes

Average cost of living

Weekly rent	● Halls £45–£90 Private £45–£55
Pint of lager	● Union Bar £1.30 City Centre pub £2
Cinema	● £1.50–£3.80
Nightclub	● £3–£9

a GP in or around Sheffield, to which students commute. First year students must shadow a patient suffering from a chronic illness, to assess the impact of disease on daily living. This is known as the Community Attachment Scheme (CAS), and takes a different approach to most of the medical course because of its emphasis on the social effects of disease rather than how to treat it.

Honours year   The option of spending an extra year studying for a BMedSci is open to anyone who has passed all their pre-clinical exams. Funding is available for most places, which are generally research laboratory based. There is little competition for places and students can 'design' their own degree. Faculty publishes a list of projects open to BMedSci students and staff tend to be very keen to recruit students.

Elective study/SSMs   There is one 8 week elective period during the fourth year. Attachments (if approved by Faculty) are usually completed abroad. Some help with funding is available.

Course organisation   Organisers of the new course are eager for student feedback and are constantly reviewing and changing the content and structure of the curriculum. Handouts outlining timetables and course objectives are provided at each stage. Formal teaching sessions are rarely cancelled. Ward teaching is more hit and miss at each stage, with some excellent and some poor teaching, depending largely on the clinician doing the teaching.

PRHO year   A large proportion of Sheffield medics stay in the locality long term. House job allocation happens in the final year, following interview and computer matching. Individual posts may include general practice and paediatrics, and last from 3 to 6 months.

The learning environment

There are four hospitals in Sheffield including the two extremely large teaching hospitals: the Northern General and the Royal Hallamshire. The other two are the Weston Park Hospital, specifically for cancer patients and the Jessops Hospital for Women. The Medical School is based at the Royal Hallamshire Hospital, which is situated right next to the main university campus. Pre-clinical teaching takes place here and in other parts of the main university site, mainly in the biomedical sciences department. The clinical years are taught on the wards of the various Sheffield and district general hospitals. Lecture blocks for the whole year group are held in the Medical School and the excellent Union cinema (!), but smaller groups attend the Northern General Hospital Education Centre. This provides much better teaching facilities, but is situated on the other side of town (20 minutes from the university).

Library facilities   Libraries are sited around the university and in all hospitals used for teaching. The two main medical libraries have been refurbished and have on-site computer access, including access to the internet and Medline. Core texts and places to sit are increasing, but be prepared to fight for them at exam time. Opening hours are reasonable, but are limited during weekends.

Computer facilities   There are widespread computer facilities throughout the university and in the Royal Hallamshire, but be prepared to wait at peak times. One site is open 24 hours. Software provided includes email, internet access, and an increasing number of computer-assisted learning packages which students are encouraged to use.

Clinical skills laboratory   There are two new labs – one at the Northern General and one at the Royal Hallamshire.

Teaching hospitals   Undergraduate common room facilities are sparse, so students tend to congregate in the hospital canteens. On-call rooms are available in Sheffield, with more permanent (free) accommodation in district general hospitals. Staff are usually friendly and willing to teach, especially in the peripheral hospitals, where its easier to pick up and practice your clinical skills.

Student friendliness and support   First year students are eased into the course fairly gently, and there are usually plenty of people around to help you with problems. Most lecturers are willing to help solve academic problems and the Undergraduate Dean is very approachable. Each student is allocated a social tutor and medical students from the years above as part of a social group to help out with any problems and offer advice, but the scheme tends to be very hit and miss, depending on the involvement of individual tutors. The scheme is currently under review. The Students Union and university have counsellors and welfare support.

Student life

Sheffield has two large universities, so there are always absolutely loads of student events taking place. The local people are generally good natured and hospitable, making it easy to settle in and fun working on the wards. Extensive redevelopment of out of town industrial areas and now the city centre has improved the range of shops, restaurants, nightclubs, cinemas and sporting facilities significantly. If you don't want to mix with the natives, Sheffield University Union is considered to be one of the best in the country, and has just been refurbished again.

If you are looking to be part of a medical clique, Sheffield may not be for you. The Sub-Dean of Admissions is keen to recruit away from the stereotypical medic, and a wide range of backgrounds are represented here. Medics are very much part of the university as a whole, and the city has such a small, friendly feel to it that settling in is quick and easy.

Accommodation   All first years are guaranteed university-owned accommodation, either in a hall of residence or self-catering. The standard is pretty good – a major plus being that it is all within easy walking distance of university and in the better part of town. Most (but not all) students move into the private rented sector for their second year. Plenty of housing is available, mostly on 12 month contracts.

Entertainment and societies   The Medical Society organises regular socials; the annual November Ball (be prepared to save up for it) and the legendary Medics Revue are particularly well supported, as well as the annual Fancy Dress Three Legged Pub Crawl and loads of lectures involving free pizza. If you would rather by pass medics after working hours, there are clubs for every type of person playing every type of music, including Gatecrasher, indie haven, The Leadmill, and the ever more popular N.Y.Sushi, while the Students Union organises cheap and cheerful events every night of the week, including Pop Tarts if you like your cheese with a high calcium content. There is a huge variety of clubs and societies available to join; anyone fancy the Assassin's Guild or the Whistling Society? Those interested in the more altruistic side to medicine can join the Marrow Appeal set up by medical students, or the Medical Students' International Network (MedSIN). In addition, people from all religious denominations are catered for through their respective religious societies.

Sports facilities   The city of Sheffield has inherited a large range of world-class sports facilities after hosting the World Student Games, including the Olympic swimming pool at Pondsforge and Don Valley athletics stadium. Unfortunately, the free university facilities are on the disappointing side; consisting mainly of a pool and several astroturf pitches. All sports are well catered for, but the dry ski slope and indoor climbing wall are particular attractions. The Medical School has numerous sports teams, with the rugby, football and hockey clubs all being active.

City and surrounds   The city centre is compact (i.e. small) and not terribly well formed, but has a good collection of small shops and restaurants, while Division Street has lots of trendy student shops. (Real shopaholics go to the purpose-built out of town Meadowhall Centre, accessible by bus, train and tram, which contains every high street store under the sun, and is the third biggest in Europe or something.) There is an ever-increasing number of new nightclubs, café-bars and live music venues. Most clubs have at least one student night a week, with cheap entry, drinks promotions, and a free bus to and from the venue. There are two theatres and five cinemas which all have student discounts for those after a bit of culture; the UGC cinema contains the biggest screen in Europe, appropriately called `The Full Monty`. The crowning glory of Sheffield is the Peak District. This attracts many active outdoor types (especially climbers) to the university, as well as those who like to chill out over a pint in a nice country pub. Just 10 minutes' drive from the university you can walk, cycle, climb, admire the stunning scenery, and forget about medicine.

The five BEST things about Sheffield Medical School

- The course allows individuals to learn things at their own pace. Lecturers are very accessible and are usually happy to help with any problems.

- The Peak District is only minutes away.

- Student accommodation is in the nicer parts of town, within easy (and safe) walking distance of the university and all local amenities.

- Sheffield medics are down to earth and represent a wide cross-section of society.

- Medical students are part of the university as a whole and not just the Medical School. This enables them to make use of all the facilities available, and escape from medicine when they want to.

The five WORST things about Sheffield Medical School

- Students complain of Faculty's lack of organisation and inability to provide up to date information on the continually changing curriculum.

- Self-directed learning is hard if you are a poor self-motivator and leave things to the last minute; with formal assessment only at the end of the year, it's easy to fall behind.

- According to the consultants, they don't teach anatomy like they used to.....or physiology, or biochemistry, etc.....

- Some of the peripheral attachments are to slightly less than glamorous towns – Hull, Grimsby, Rotherham, Scunthorpe and Barnsley etc.

- Hills – good practice if you're training for Everest.

Further information

Admissions: Sub-Dean for Admissions
Medical School
University of Sheffield
Beech Hill Road
Sheffield
S10 2RX
Tel: 0114 271 1910
Fax: 0114 271 3961 or 3960

Southampton

The Medical School at Southampton University is modern and student-friendly It is one of the youngest medical schools, with a well-developed modern course. Southampton pioneered the new integrated curriculum now in operation in most UK medical schools. As such it has had more experience than most schools at settling in to the new ways of learning medicine. Plans exist to develop an innovative programme of interprofessional learning in conjunction with the School of Nursing and Midwifery and the School of Health Professions and Rehabilitation Sciences. Southampton has just about everything city life has to offer but on a scale which is easy to cope with and, of course, it's by the sea!

The course

The fully integrated course has an increasing clinical component throughout the 5 years. During the first 2 years, each term deals with the basic science and clinical aspects of a major organ system, and includes clinical sessions in general practice and in the labour ward. Year 3 is the first clinical year, and students work in the Southampton area. Exams at the end of this year integrate basic science and clinical knowledge, a feature which is valued by students. The fourth year comprises clinical experience in the minor specialties, plus a research project. This educational innovation enables students to study an area of their choice for 8 months, finishing with a dissertation and presentation. Some are fascinated by their project, whilst others are not and feel they forget a lot of the first 3 years' teaching. Final year students are spread throughout the Wessex region in large teaching hospitals and smaller district general hospitals.

Southampton has complied with GMC recommendations to limit the factual knowledge which is required, and, as a result, the examinations are not structured to make you regurgitate thousands of facts but to test your ability to solve clinical problems (i.e. be a good doctor!).

Teaching and assessment   In the early years students spend most of their time on the main university campus with other, non-medical, students learning in lectures, tutorials and laboratory practicals. The major exams are at the end of years 1 and 3 and throughout the final year. Anatomy at Southampton is taught in a small department from pre-dissected cadavers, reflecting the lack of emphasis on regurgitation of facts. Southampton students have a reputation amongst old-style consultants for not knowing their anatomy; however, there is no concrete evidence that students suffer by this teaching method. Southampton is introducing computer-based learning into the curriculum, although this is not yet a major part of any area of the course.

Placements outside the university Final year clinical attachments may be in local Southampton hospitals or as far afield as Bath or Basingstoke. With no other medical schools in the region, there are fewer students per hospital and, consequently, more individual attention; students give excellent feedback from these placements. Accommodation and travel expenses are provided on peripheral attachments.

Course details

Course length	● 5 years
Total number of medical undergraduates	● c. 800
Male/Female ratio	● n/a

Admission procedure

Average A level requirements	● AAB Must include Chemistry and one other Science
Average Scottish Higher requirements	● Please check with Southampton
Number of applicants (Sept 2000 entry)	● c. 2500
Proportion of applicants interviewed	● Only mature and overseas applicants are interviewed
Make up of interview panel	● Academic, clinician and lay person
Months interviews held	● Throughout the year
Number admitted (Sept 2000 entry)	● c. 180
Proposed entry size for 2001	● 200
Proportion of overseas students	● 12 per intake
Proportion of mature students	● 25 per intake
Faculty's view of taking a gap year	● Acceptable if used for work experience, voluntary service or travel
Proportion taking Intercalated Hons	● 15%
Possibility of direct entrance to clinical phase	● No

Finances

Tuition fees per year	● £1050
Fees for self-funding students	● £1050
Fees for graduates	● £1050
Fees for overseas students	● £9050 p.a. (pre-clinical) and £17 540 p.a. (clinical)
Assistance for elective funding	● Limited bursaries available
Assistance for travel to attachments	● Under review
Access and hardship funds	● Yes

Average cost of living

Weekly rent	● Halls £42–£93 Private £45
Pint of lager	● Union Bar £1.40 City Centre pub £2
Cinema	● £2–£5
Nightclub	● Free–£8

Honours year   Between 5% and 15% of students take the opportunity to spend an extra year between third and fourth year to study for a BSc in basic or social sciences. Only a few students opt for the extra year because of the extra financial expense of another year as a student, and because all students spend time in research during the fourth year. Students who already have undergraduate research experience may skip the fourth year project and take an accelerated course, qualifying 6 months earlier.

Elective study/SSMs   At the end of the third year students have an 8 week elective during which they may decide to spend time working in a hospital abroad. There are Special Study Modules during the third year, where students may choose to study a particular area in depth, and in the fifth year there is a 5 week block when students choose which specialty to gain additional experience in.

Course organisation   Students are asked for feedback on every aspect of the course and changes can be achieved. More often than not the changes reflect the student feedback (but not always). Students sit on co-ordinating bodies for each year of the course; these bodies develop the delivery of the curriculum from year to year.

PRHO year   The Medical School operates a matching scheme which guarantees all Southampton graduates a PRHO job in the Wessex region. Most, but by no means all, students get at least one of their two preferred PRHO jobs, but there's always someone who has to go to the Isle of Wight in the winter!

The learning environment

The main university campus is in the Highfield/Bassett area of Southampton and is close to most of the halls of residence. The General Hospital where most of the third and fourth years are spent is about 1 mile away in Shirley. There is a reliable university bus service connecting all sites.

Library facilities   Students have access to the Biomedical Sciences Library on the main campus and the Health Sciences Library at the General Hospital. Library facilities are good, although the most popular texts are always in demand and students find it more convenient to buy core books.

Computer facilities   The computer facilities are very good and are updated regularly. Workstations are available all over the campus, at the General Hospital, and in some halls of residence.

Clinical skills laboratory   This is operational, but so far has had limited impact on students. Things are getting better.

Teaching hospitals   Southampton General and the Royal South Hampshire are the two main teaching hospitals. Hospitals further afield are used increasingly in the later years. These locations include Portsmouth, Bournemouth, and Salisbury.

Student friendliness and support   Most people are struck by the friendliness of the staff and students at the Medical School when they visit. A scheme has been set up recently where students run mini-tutorials for younger students in order to pass on the most relevant information: which books to buy, books not to buy, consultants with nice yachts who often need crew on trips round the Channel Isles – all the really important stuff. Southampton University has a counselling service and the Students Union has welfare services.

Student life

As an integral part of a big university, medical students live and work with other students and have access to a wide range of sports and social facilities. Southampton isn't the Mecca of UK nightlife, but with an enormous student population it has enough to keep most energetic party animals occupied. Somehow it manages to keep its football team in the premiership.

Accommodation   Students will be offered a place in halls of residence for their first year only. There's a range of options, from a small self-catering room with no sink, to a large en suite room with breakfast and evening meal. Which one to choose is mostly governed by your bank balance! A limited number of places are available in halls for subsequent years, but most people move into private rented houses in the Highfield and Portswood areas. Most Halls are within a mile of the Medical School.

Entertainment and societies   The Students Union runs every club you could ever imagine wanting to join, and quite a few others besides! The Students Union building hosts nightclub events and bands. The on-site theatre and concert hall host lots of non-mainstream acts and performances. The Medical School is renowned for its strong social life, and has a number of sporting and other societies. There is an annual ball, which is the most popular in the university, and an extravagant Christmas revue, which never fails to entertain.

Sports facilities   The University of Southampton has excellent water sports teams. The facilities are accessible to those who have never sailed/rowed/canoed in their lives, ranging up to those who wish to compete at an international level. At the moment the facilities aren't great for outdoor sports or swimming, but Southampton has teams in most sports.

City and surrounds   Southampton itself is not a particularly attractive town, having been heavily bombed during the war and subjected to the worst aspects of modern rebuilding. There is a wide range of shops and restaurants, and most of the amenities you would expect of a city are evident. The New Forest is popular for nature lovers, cyclists and "pub-lunchers", and the Solent and the Isle of Wight are popular with sailors. The proximity to Bournemouth beach is a bonus for sun and sand lovers. London is close enough for a day or night out by car or train.

The five BEST things about Southampton Medical School

- Excellent course which is well-liked by students.

- Good patient/doctor to student ratio on attachments.

- Students are part of the main university not just the Medical School.

- Southampton General Hospital is an excellent, friendly place to train.

- It's the furthest south of UK Medical Schools and, therefore, the warmest – and it's by the sea!

The five WORST things about Southampton Medical School

- Being one of the newest medical schools, some of the older consultants tend to be sceptical about any "new-fangled" ways of doing things.

- No astroturf pitches or swimming pool.

- The city's nightlife isn't what it could be.

- Having the elective after just one year of clinical work makes you less useful in a hospital abroad.

- Some of the fifth year attachments can leave you feeling isolated and away from Southampton (for example Swindon, Dorchester), but this doesn't last too long.

Further information

Admissions: Admissions Office
University of Southampton
Biomedical Sciences Building
Bassett Crescent East
Southampton
SO15 7FX
Tel: 01703 594 408
Fax: 01703 594 159

Wales (Cardiff)

The University of Wales College of Medicine in Cardiff is a member college of the University of Wales responsible for the provision of teaching of medicine, dentistry, nursing, radiography, physiotherapy, occupational therapy, and other professions allied to medicine. This provides a unique Students Union solely for these students. The university has strong links with all hospitals in Wales, offering clinical placements across the principality. Students from all walks of life – mature, overseas, Welsh, non-Welsh, and even resit students – make a varied student body, providing a peer group for almost any person. The university is ideally located for the leisure/recreation/social facilities available in this small, yet friendly capital city.

The course

The course has been following the new curriculum since October 1995. The new course is guided by five themes and delivered through 11 subject panels, with practical experience gained through clinical modules. Year 1 is the foundation year, introducing basic clinical and scientific skills and knowledge, with years 2 and 3 developing further the scientific principles and clinical skills. Years 4 and 5 place a greater emphasis on clinical experience in preparing for housemanship. Teaching is provided through core and Special Study Modules components.

Teaching and assessment   A combination of lectures, tutorials, small-group sessions and self-directed learning make up the bulk of the learning. Some animal experiments are still conducted, but participation is optional. Anatomy is taught using demonstrated dissection and prosections. Various computer-assisted learning programs are used mainly as a revision medium and for tutorial support. Firm sizes vary depending on the hospital: five to six in the main teaching hospitals, and usually two in the DGHs (varying from one to four). Examinations take place at the end of 1st, 3rd, 4th and 5th years. Continuous assessment and the satisfactory completion of all coursework and Special Study Modules is a feature of the examination process.

Placements outside the university   All NHS hospitals within Wales are used for teaching attachments. Attachments in general practice include some time spent at a rural practice somewhere in Wales. Travel subsidies are available from the college, and accommodation is provided in all DGHs.

Honours year   Intercalated degrees are available to one-third of the year, and can be done after years 2, 3 and 4. There is a choice of subjects, including basic medical sciences (anatomy, physiology, biochemistry), or more clinically orientated, modular degrees in medical sciences.

Elective study/SSMs   An 8 week period of elective study, either in the UK or abroad, is undertaken in the final year as part of the normal block rotation. Special Study Modules make up 30–40% of the timetable.

Course details

Course length	● 5 years
Total number of medical undergraduates	● 989
Male/Female ratio	● 43:57

Admission procedure

Average A level requirements	● AAB Chemistry and Biology (preferred) or physics plus one other – not General Studies)
Average Scottish Higher requirements	● AAAAB (including Chemistry, Biology, Physics and English) and 2 advanced Highers AA including Chemstriy
Number of applicants (Sept 2000 entry)	● 1300
Proportion of applicants interviewed	● 50%
Make up of interview panel	● Mix of clinicians, GPs and Scientists, lay people, staff in medically related fields (radiography, nursing etc) + medical students
Months interviews held	● November–March
Number admitted (Sept 2000 entry)	● 230
Proposed entry size for 2001	● 290
Proportion of overseas students	● 10%
Proportion of mature students	● 6%
Faculty's view of taking a gap year	● Happy to consider applicants for deferred entry provided the year is spent constructively
Proportion taking Intercalated Hons	● 20–33%
Possibility of direct entrance to clinical phase	● There must be strong personal reasons to transfer in and courses must be compatible

Finances

Tuition fees per year	● £1050
Fees for self-funding students	● £1050
Fees for graduates	● £1050
Fees for overseas students	● £9 000 p.a. (pre-clinical) and £16 600 p.a. (clinical)
Assistance for elective funding	● Some small scholarships available
Assistance for travel to attachments	● Free transport provided in South Wales area 50% of rail fare to mid/North Wales
Access and hardship funds	● Emergency loan funds and some grants available

Average cost of living

Weekly rent	● Halls £35 Private £40
Pint of lager	● Union Bar £1.30 City Centre pub £1.90
Cinema	● £3–£4.50
Nightclub	● Free–£5

Course organisation The course is well organised, supported by a comprehensive document given to all students charting the forthcoming year. There is a limited amount of choice in the location of peripheral hospital attachments.

PRHO year Allocation of jobs is by an internal application system run by the postgraduate department. There are sufficient PRHO posts available within the scheme (for all posts in Wales) to accommodate all UWCM graduates. The system is a computer matching scheme, matching students' preferred choices with those of consultants. Students are able to apply outside Wales for PRHO posts.

The learning environment

The Medical School is based on two sites, the School of Molecular and Medical Biosciences (a part of University of Wales, Cardiff) and UWCM at the University Hospital of Wales, the two sites being approximately 1.5 miles apart. Community-based teaching is in practices in and around Cardiff, and this forms a substantial part of the course. Clinical teaching takes place in hospitals throughout Wales.

Library facilities The library facilities in the main teaching hospital consist of three separate libraries, two 24 hour reading rooms and a 40 PC 24 hour computer room. The availability of texts and journals is excellent. Students also have access to the library and computing facilities of the University of Wales, Cardiff, and many other libraries in most hospitals.

Computer facilities There are adequate computer facilities on site and within most outlying hospitals. Some tuition is initially given, and all submitted work is expected to be word processed.

Clinical skills laboratory Cardiff has a new skills laboratory which is used heavily. It is a key focus for the new curriculum.

Teaching hospitals Hospitals throughout Wales are utilised for teaching, ensuring a good student–patient ratio. It also provides an opportunity for students to see all of the various sites and sides of Wales.

Student friendliness and support UWCM is very student friendly and actively encourages and acts upon the views of its students. Monthly meetings between year reps and the Dean occur where students' grievances are voiced in an informal setting. Students are also represented on all the curriculum planning committees. Being part of the University of Wales allows students access to its general counselling and welfare services. These resources may feel a little remote for medics, particularly in the latter years, but most pastoral needs can be met within the Faculty.

Student life

Student life can be very hectic, juggling work commitments with the variety of sports and clubs offered by UWCM Students Club. The majority of teams, clubs and societies are fully funded by the Club, including the provision of three minibuses for the use of its members. Its own bar/club provides a friendly/social/cheap venue for the post-match celebrations. It also provides a very cheap source of alcohol for those not partaking in the sporting scene! The Students Club also has a multigym, pool and snooker tables. Besides the facilities on offer by the dedicated Students Union of UWCM, students have the benefit of using the sports and Union facilities of University of Wales, Cardiff. As a capital city, Cardiff also offers excellent sport, leisure and recreational facilities. The new Millenium Stadium has opened recently and has hosted the Rugby World Cup and hosted the FA Cup and Worthington Cup Finals in 2001.

Accommodation   Accommodation is provided in the first two years by the University of Wales. There is normally space for all first years in halls. The standards are high, with over 50% of accommodation being less than 5 years old. There is ample good quality private housing for rent, with prices ranging from £35 to £45 a week. Cardiff Council runs a house renting registration scheme, which aims to monitor and license rented accommodation in the city.

Entertainment and societies   Medical students are members of their own Students Club which provides members with sporting facilities/teams, its own fleet of minibuses and its own bar, where drinks are often the cheapest in Cardiff! The Students Club organises three staff/student dinners a year, six balls and many other social events, ranging from top-name bands, comedians, long distance pub crawls and tours around the UK – all attended by a mix of medics, dentists, nurses, radiographers and physiotherapy students. A range of activities, including choir, orchestra, chess and photography are available, in addition to the usual clubs and societies. A charity revue is staged in the third year. Students also have access to the much greater facilities provided by the University of Wales, Cardiff, and its Students Union.

Sports facilities   The Club has a large number of teams, many of which gain great success, far beyond that expected of a small university. Most teams compete in the various BUSA inter-university competitions, inter-medical school competitions, as well as some local leagues.

City and surrounds   Cardiff is a very student friendly city. UWCM, UW Cardiff, UW Institute Cardiff and the Welsh College of Music and Drama combine to make a student population of over 20 000. Most clubs/pubs/theatres etc. host student nights/special rates for NUS card holders. The city also has plenty of parks and open spaces, so there is always somewhere to relax, especially in the summer. As the capital, Cardiff has all the attractions that you would expect of a large city, while being small enough to make you feel at home. The local countryside is very beautiful, and all outdoor activities are available. The Welsh Assembly has given added excitement to the atmosphere in the city.

The five BEST things about Cardiff Medical School

- Great staff/student relationship.
- A lot of interactions (socially and academically!) between all students of all years, and dental, nursing, physios, etc. and students are members of the Students Union at UWCC (Cardiff Uni) and UWCM.
- A friendly university located in a student-friendly city.
- Using all Welsh hospitals keeps firm sizes low and student/patient ratio high.
- Rugby mad!

The five WORST things about Cardiff Medical School

- The large year group size means it can be difficult to get to know all fellow students individually.
- Course-work deadlines and exams all come at the same time.

- Distances between hospitals and accessibility of some rural hospitals makes travelling very awkward/time-consuming, unless you have a car.

- In Wales it always rains. Rain that clearly soaks you and rain that soaks you without you realising it.

- Rugby mad.

Further information

Admissions: Undergraduate Admissions Officer
University of Wales College of Medicine
Heath Park
Cardiff
CF4 4XN
Tel: 029 2074 2027
Fax. 029 2074 2914

Medical Schools in London (University of London)

Studying medicine in London

Many prospective medics will consider applying to one or more of the London medical schools. Some might dismiss the idea quickly, and others might apply without really thinking about the possible differences that studying in London involves. If you do have anxieties about being a medical student in London, they probably fall into one of two categories: London is too big and very unfriendly, or, it will cost too much to live in London. The London medics who have helped us write the Guide would not want you to be put off by either of these worries.

Is London an unfriendly place? No. London is a large place and possibly a daunting prospect to anyone who hasn't previously lived in the centre of a large city. However, Londoners are no more friendly or less friendly than anyone else. You will be starting your course with 100+ other students and many of them will be living in London for the first time too. Student unions, medsocs and medical schools should all be familiar with the kinds of problems moving to London as a student can cause. There is a range of people you can turn to for advice and support.

Is London expensive? Yes and No. London can be very expensive, but cheap nights out and affordable living do exist. It may take a bit of finding but it is out there, and if you budget sensibly you will cope. On average, medical students in London do have a higher burden of debt than medics at other schools, despite getting slightly higher student loans. Many students work at weekends and during vacations, although there is less opportunity to do this in the clinical years. However, it is possible to survive on a maintenance loan plus some extra income, and, although the vast majority of medics have a financial struggle, it is only a tiny minority who find the struggle too much.

London has much to offer the medical student. A glance at the weekly *Time Out* will give an impression of just how much there is to do. All the schools have good facilities and social calendars as well as their own thriving medical societies. Some schools are the product of mergers, and all of the medical schools – with the exception of St George's – are linked within multi-disciplinary colleges. These generally have a wide range of sports teams and societies, as well as libraries and bars, to supplement those in the medical schools. All London medics are also members of the University of London and have access to the services (including a pool and very well-equipped sports facility) and the societies of the Union (ULU) in Bloomsbury. Medical student representation thus takes place at three levels: the school, the "parent" college and ULU.

Students with an intercalated BSc qualification or equivalent may apply to the clinical courses at Oxford or Cambridge in their 3rd year. However, it is interesting to note that the greater movement is out of these institutions into London.

Of course, every medical school and every town and city has a lot to be said for it, and we are not suggesting that London is better or worse than anywhere else. We hope the Guide will give you a flavour of what each of the medical schools has to offer. After that, it's up to you.

London is a very big city and the medical schools are in different parts of the capital. Nowhere in central London is far from fine open spaces (Regent's Park, Hampstead Heath, Tooting Bec Common, Dulwich Common, Hyde Park, etc.) and getting around on public transport is normally, easy. All the schools are near to underground stations (although the King's College Hospital site is a little distance from the Victoria Line) and overland trains and bus routes are numerous. Outside London students tend to rent private accommodation in particular areas. The sheer size of the city and the range of public transport allow London students to search widely for the best available accommodation and commuting into the school from another part of London, or travelling across London, is not uncommon. You are as likely to live in Ealing, Haringey, Wembley, Streatham, Kentish Town, New Cross or the Isle of Dogs at some stage during your studies as you are to live on the doorstep of the medical school.

To help you distinguish between the schools, we have the put the City and Surrounds sections together below. We apologise if information is repeated in the profiles.

Guy's, King's and St Thomas'
The three hospital campuses for GKT are south of the river. The two campuses near to the Thames – St Thomas' Hospital which looks across the river to the Houses of Parliament and Westminster, and Guy's near London Bridge, with great views over the city – put you at London's doorstep. The West End, Oxford Street, the Tower of London, the South Bank, the City and Whitehall are all within walking distance of one or both of the sites. King's College Hospital campus is in Denmark Hill, Camberwell, part of the south London sprawl of inner city and suburbia. From here you can get to Brixton very easily with its market, clubs and cafes, and you are still not far from central London. King's College London has a campus on the Strand, just north of, and overlooking, the River Thames.

Accommodation in halls is normally close to the hospitals, but some University of London halls will be elsewhere in the city. Many students live in Denmark Hill/Camberwell in the later years, and accommodation there is less expensive than around the more central Guy's and St Thomas'.

Imperial
Imperial College is in West Kensington near the big museums (Natural History, V&A, Science Museum) and the Royal Albert Hall. Transport to the rest of central London is good, with a variety of tubes and buses running to the West End. The hospitals are in Paddington (St Mary's) and Hammersmith (Charing Cross and Westminster). These are bustling areas of inner London with shops, cinemas, theatres, etc., all within a short bus journey. Paddington and Hammersmith are not the most glamorous of neighbourhoods, but they do not have the accommodation price tags that accompany more exclusive addresses.

Royal Free and University College Medical School
The Royal Free is based in Hampstead which, although surrounded by London, maintains a village type feel. There are plenty of pubs, cafes and restaurants (where you can go "luvvie" spotting). Hampstead Heath provides, amongst other things, a large open space, summer football, baseball, picnics, parties and winter sledging. University College is in Bloomsbury, adjacent to the West End, Covent Garden and theatreland. There is no mistaking that you are at the heart of a big city. Students living near to either site can expect to pay higher rents, but cheaper areas are reasonably close. Camden Town is full of buzz with the market and clubs.

Bart's and the Royal London (QMW)

The medical school's three sites are in the City and East End of London. The East End has traditionally been home to immigrant communities and suffers serious deprivation. With the local Asian and Muslim populations, the markets and shops are colourful and Brick Lane has the cheapest and best curries in the capital. It isn't all poverty, and Old Street and Clerkenwell are very up and coming in terms of fashionable bars and restaurants. Greenwich is just a short journey away, and there are good public transport services to get into central and west London. Of all the London medical schools, Bart's and the Royal London has easiest access to affordable accommodation.

St George's

St George's is the London medical school furthest away from the city centre. It is situated in Tooting, south London. There is easy access to central London by underground train (up the Northern line), and the normal journey time is 20 minutes. Tooting has its own high street and lots of reasonably priced accommodation (by London standards). St George's is part of the University of London, but only offers healthcare courses (medicine and nursing, etc.). This makes it the smallest of the London medical schools. It is easy to get into London from St George's, but most students will focus their social lives around Tooting, Wandsworth, Wimbledon and Clapham, with their wide range of clubs, pubs, cafes, cinemas and restaurants.

Medical Schools in London
(University of London)

Guy's, King's and St Thomas'

King's College School of Medicine and Dentistry (KCSMD) and the United Medical and Dental School (UMDS) of Guy's and St Thomas' Hospitals merged in August 1998 to form part of King's College London. The new college is popularly known as GKT, to avoid yet another mouthful (the full title is the Guy's, King's and St Thomas' School of Medicine). The first joint intake started in 1999 and has so far gone well.

This new school combines two established medical schools both with long histories including older mergers. King's College is a multi-disciplinary institution, part of the university of London and had its own medical school at King's College Hospital in South London. Guy's and St Thomas' Hospitals had their own medical schools prior to a very recent merger to form the United Medical and Dental Schools. An intake of over 360 students makes the new school a very large creature and it is one of the biggest medical schools in Europe. Both King's and UMDS emphasised personal academic development (e.g. a strongly supported intercalated BSc programme) and encouraged students to participate fully in extracurricular activities. This is still a strong feature of the new GKT.

The course

The curricula at the two schools have been streamlined over the last few years as part of the preparation for the merger, and will, therefore, not be brand new (but there remains potential for teething problems). The course is split into two main sections. The first two years place an emphasis on the basic medical sciences. Clinical contact is rare in these years, except during communications exercises. The course is organised into systems based study focusing on for example the cardiovascular system or the musculoskeletal system. The majority of students appear to find this a more useful way of learning. A disadvantage, however, is that many textbooks concentrate on specific subject areas such as biochemistry or anatomy and it is sometimes necessary to look at up to four books at the same time when studying. All the core basic science teaching takes place at the Guy's Hospital Campus.

Clinical disciplines are taught in the latter 3 years, on the wards of St Thomas' Hospital, King's College Hospital, Guy's Hospital, Lewisham Hospital and also in the community. A new systems-based clinical course has been designed and was introduced in 1988 to complement the course structure from the earlier years. The core clinical subjects are delivered and examined during years 3 and 4. The final year

Course Details

Course length	● 5 years
Total number of undergraduates	● 1942
Male/Female ratio	● 47:53

Admission Procedure

Average A level requirements	● ABB including Chemistry + Biology at GCSE B grade at first sitting
Average Scottish Higher requirements	● CSYS ABB
Number of applicants (Sept 2000 entry)	● 3700
Proportion of applicants interviewed	● 33%
Make-up of interview panel	● 1 clinical and 1 pre-clinical member of staff +/– observer from local schools
Months interviews held	● Nov–March
Number admitted (Sept 2000 entry)	● 359
Proposed intake for 2002	● 387
Proportion of overseas students	● 27 (Quota)
Proportion of mature students	● c. 9%
Faculty's view of taking a gap year	● Encouraged if spent well, and is clear what they are going to achieve
Proportion taking Intercalated Hons	● 50%
Possibility of direct entrance to clinical phase	● Yes, especially Oxbridge and those achieving at least a 2:1 in Medical Sciences at Leeds University

Finances

Fees for self-funding students	● £1050 p.a.
Fees for graduates	● £1050 p.a.
Fees for overseas students	● £10 375 p.a. (pre-clinical) and £19 250 p.a. (clinical)
Assistance for elective funding	● Students may compete for limited funds
Assistance for travel to attachments	● No, only for peripheral attachment in Obstetrics and Gynaecology where 1 return journey is paid for.
Access and hardship funds	● Available

Average Cost of Living

Weekly rent	● Halls £85 (inc. food and bills) Private £40–£80
Pint of lager	● Union £1.30–£1.50 City Centre pub £2–£2.20
Cinema	● £2.50 (local) £15 West End
Night-club	● Free–£20

consists of an 8 week elective followed by attachments in the community in general practice settings, and attachments shadowing house officers in district general hospitals.

Stop press

King's College London (KCL) has recently secured funding for an exciting new programme working with local schools to widen the social and ethnic mix of medical students. The following is a press statement (dated 16 June 2000) from KCL about the Access to Medicine programme.

Major initiative to widen access to medicine

In a major initiative to widen access to medical degree courses, King's College London is launching Access to Medicine, a programme specifically designed to help bright and talented young people from disadvantaged backgrounds to become doctors. The programme will be announced by the Prime Minister during a speech today.

The programme will eventually allow for up to 50 **extra** undergraduate places in medicine and will be for talented school pupils from south London who would not normally achieve the necessary grades to train as doctors.

King's College London includes the medical and dental schools of Guy's, King's and St Thomas' Hospitals, and is the largest centre for medical education in Europe. The new programme is ground-breaking in that selection criteria will be based on pupil potential rather than A Level grades; this alternative route of entry to medicine will entail equally rigorous assessment procedures devised by the renowned School of Education of King's College.

The pilot programme will evolve through partnerships with local schools and Sixth Form colleges to provide:
- Early identification of students with potential to learn (from Year 9 onwards) through work with students and parents.
- 'Science in action' sessions on the medical school campus and teacher placements on the medical school campus.
- Joint development of appropriate project work in schools.
- Work observation and experience schemes at Guy's, St. Thomas', Lewisham and King's College Hospital.
- Mentoring by medical school staff, medical students, and the students themselves as they progress through the course.

Ten additional medical students per year will be accepted for the access programme from August 2001, rising to 50 per year from 2006. The course is based on a standard MBBS course but will take six years rather than five years because of the addition of special modules in the first three years. In the final clinical year, partnership with the University of Kent at Canterbury will provide placements in hospitals and GP practices in Kent.

King's Vice Principal Sir Cyril Chantler said: "This new programme is the result of two years' planning and offers a completely new approach to providing equal opportunities for all in our society."

For more details about the Access course please contact GKT undergraduate admissions office: Tel 020 7848 6501 Email: gktadmissions@kcl.ac.uk

---

Teaching and assessment There is a mixture of lectures, tutorials and practicals, mixed in with computer-assisted learning. Essays, SAQ's, MCQs, OSCEs and vivas are all used for assessment. Written examinations during the clinical years are now mostly computer marked, and offer some element of choice in the answer. Essay and short answer questions are now rare during years 3 to 5, as there is a move towards more MCQ-based format. Negative marking for wrong answers in MCQ exams has been abolished.

Placements outside the university As well as use of the central teaching hospitals, in years 4 and 5, there are placements in DGHs in south east England. This relieves some of the pressures at the central London teaching hospitals and provides access to high quality teaching, because clinical workloads tend to be lower and consultants are able to devote more time to students.

Honours year There are well-supported intercalated degree programmes at the college, and around 60-70% of students are expected to take an intercalated BSc. There is a wide range of options, including many outside the sciences and medicine, to choose from.

Elective study The 8 week elective period is an opportunity to travel to far flung destinations (or just down the road) to do clerkships in fields of medicine of your choosing. There is some assessment of how time is spent on the elective (to discourage the temptation to just lie on a beach for 8 weeks), and at the moment this is in the form of a poster presentation. Various awards and sponsorships are available to help students fund their electives. The school has special links with numerous medical schools around the world including The Johns Hopkins University in the USA, the University of Hong Kong, the University of West Indies and Moscow Medical Academy. As GKT is twinned with these institutions, there are special allocations for GKT students who want to do their electives there. Accommodation will also usually be arranged for you, and extra bursaries may be available to help with travel costs to these colleges.

Special Study Modules About 20% of each year is devoted to SSMs. There is a considerable range of subjects available and the number of these is increasing every year. Being part of a multi-faculty institution, there are also many non-medical SSMs available, such as a choice of modern languages. Students may also design their own SSMs if the subject they wish to study is not on offer.

PRHO Year A matching scheme for PRHO posts on campus exists that is based on the ranking of students on a league table. Ranking is based on academic performance during the course, contribution to college life, and research accomplishments. There is no interview. For posts at district general hospitals from further afield, there is separate scheme with an interview.

The learning environment

Students in years 1 and 2 are taught at the newly developed Guy's Hospital campus at London Bridge. The campus is shared with other departments in the Biomedical Sciences and Nursing Schools. Most of the Guy's site has been refurbished to accommodate the large numbers of students and many facilities are new. In particular a large new building has been erected that houses most of the above disciplines, with state of the art library and computing facilities. Most of the clinical teaching takes place at King's College Hospital, St Thomas' Hospital, Guy's Hospital and University Hospital, Lewisham.

Students can also access King's College's other campuses including the Strand campus. Guy's, St Thomas' and the Strand campuses are all situated within a square mile on both sides of the Thames in central London.

Library facilities   Guy's Library is open between 9 a.m. and 8.45 p.m. on weekdays, 9 a.m. and 4.45 p.m. on Saturday, and 1 p.m. and 4.45 p.m. on Sunday. At the Denmark Hill campus, the library is open until 9 p.m. on weekdays, and 1 p.m. on Saturday. Students also have access to King's College Library, which is open until 9 p.m. from Monday to Thursday, 6 p.m. on Friday, and 5.30 p.m. on Saturday. All libraries have a good range of books and journals.

Computer facilities   All campuses have computer stations with access to email, the internet, and some in-house designed computer-assisted learning programmes. There are 24 hour computing facilities at Guy's, and late/weekend opening at the St Thomas' campus.

The "virtual campus" has also been launched this year. This is a specialised area of the King's College website for the Schools of Medicine, Dentistry and Biomedical Sciences and enables students to do things like download lecture notes, register for course components or obtain details (but not the answers) about their exams.

Clinical skills laboratory   There are labs at the three main hospitals. These are great places with latex models of every imaginable part of the human anatomy on which students can practise their clinical skills such as taking blood pressure or suturing (in the past, King's students on accident and emergency attachments practised suturing pigs' trotters before being let loose on the population of South London!). A new centre opened on the Guy's campus in 1999. It is the largest of its kind in Europe, and is available every weekday from 9 a.m. to 5 p.m. Students can book individual rooms in small groups or with their tutor.

Teaching hospitals   The main teaching hospitals will be King's College Hospital (at Denmark Hill, South London), Guy's Hospital (London Bridge), St Thomas' Hospital (Westminster) and the University Hospital, Lewisham. Psychiatry teaching happens at the Maudsley Hospital and other institutions in South London.

Student friendliness and support   New students are assigned to a personal tutor to support them throughout the course. Welfare and counselling services are available on the Guy's campus, where there is an on-site Welfare Officer available everyday. All sites are friendly environments with lots of support from the faculty and staff.

There is also the Student Medical Education Committee (SMEC), which is a unique, student-run audit committee that is actively involved in course development and provides feedback to course organisers on how things are going. It acts as a dedicated link between the medical school and the student body. There are six representatives in each year, and they will help students to deal with any problems that arise with the course and address any associated welfare concerns.

Student life

The new GKT medical school gives students access to a large multi-disciplinary institution while retaining the friendliness of a medical school. The mix of students on a day-to-day basis may not be diverse, but as students use King's College and University of London Union facilities, there will be plenty of opportunity for integration. Most of the campuses are close to the centre of London, with all of London's attractions within easy reach by public transport.

Accommodation   University accommodation will be guaranteed for one of the 5 years of the course, but not necessarily for the first year. College accommodation is available in many different parts of London. Some residences may be on or near the campuses themselves (on site accommodation is available on the Guy's and St Thomas' campus), whilst others may be much further away. The quality and cost of private accommodation can vary a lot in the central Guy's/St Thomas' area, but cheaper, good quality accommodation is more readily available in the Denmark Hill area. Students can opt for Intercollegiate University of London accommodation instead, although these tend to be some distance from any of the campuses.

Entertainment and societies   The old colleges always had thriving social scenes, with numerous balls, weekly discos, the annual revues and rag week. The traditions have all continued after the merger and as the college grows, more exciting developments are expected. There is a vast selection of clubs and societies to join, and everyone can usually find something that interests them. The Student Union is based on the Guy's campus, where a new nightclub and bar was built in 1999. Student bars are present on all campuses, and there is also another college nightclub at the Strand campus. If all that's not enough, all students have access to the University of London Union (ULU) with its own range of facilities.

Sports facilities   Rugby union, football, hockey, netball, tennis, rowing and squash are particularly strong. GKT has sports grounds at Honor Oak Park in South London, Cobham in Surrey and Dulwich, giving facilities for rugby, football and hockey. King's College also has sports grounds in Surbiton. There are gyms at the Guy's and St Thomas' campuses and also at the Stamford Street halls of residence. For the swimmers, there is a pool at Guy's. There is also a pool and gym at ULU.

The five BEST things about GKT Medical School

- The new school is part of a multi-faculty institution. Students will have the opportunity to mix with a variety of students from other courses, and have access to a wide range of facilities.

- GKT hospitals are all world-renowned.

- Excellent range of learning and social facilities with more on the way.

- Good sports clubs (some with lots of history).

- Welfare and student support mechanisms are well established and are effective.

The five WORST things about GKT Medical School

- Cost of living in London.

- Large number of medics in each year group can lead to it being a bit impersonal.

- Split-site arrangements leads to some inconvenience when moving around.

- The medical school can be a bit bureaucratic.

- Student accommodation can be a long way from your campus.

Further information

Admissions: Student Admissions Officer
The Hodgkin Building
Guy's Hospital Campus
King's College London
St Thomas' Street
London Bridge
London
SE1 9RT
Tel: 020 7848 6501/6511   Fax: 020 7848 6510

Imperial

Imperial College School of Medicine is the product of a merger between Charing Cross and Westminster School of Medicine and St Mary's School of Medicine. The first intake on the new course began in autumn 1998. There is full integration between the parent medical schools. Imperial College School of Medicine has created a new identity, whilst maintaining the spirit and traditions of the original schools. Initial problems created by the merger and new course appear to have been sorted out. Research at both medical schools has traditionally been strong, and this has been aided by incorporation into Imperial College. There is a new building (The Sir Alexander Fleming building) at the Imperial College site in South Kensington, which is very central and only 100m from Hyde Park. Halls of residence are close to this site. Imperial is now one of the largest medical schools in the country, and the non-course elements (such as sport and music) are flourishing in their new environment.

The course

It is a 6 year course, which incorporates an intercalated Honours year for everyone except appropriately qualified graduates who may apply for an exemption. (Mature student non-graduates are expected to undertake 6 years.) There is integrated teaching from day 1, which includes early ward exposure and general practice experience. There is a term-based structure for the first and second years (see prospectus). A wide variety of clinical experience is offered, at many sites. The course takes advantage of the large number of hospitals relatively near to Imperial. New courses are being introduced, including a business course and "introduction to graduate medical practice".

Teaching and assessment A mixture of exams and continuous assessment is used to monitor students' progress. Problem-based learning in small groups is a key feature of the teaching at Imperial. Students are encouraged to use computers and clinical skills labs. Lectures and ward attachments occur during all parts of the course, but as you progress more time is spent in hospital attachments. Anatomy is taught from the second year by dissection of cadavers. However, a shift towards using pre-dissected models will continue.

Placements outside the university Students experience a wide range of clinical attachments, starting with a GP practice in the first year. Many attachments will be near to Imperial College. However, occasionally they will be much further afield, such as Cornwall or Scotland. Free hospital accommodation is nearly always provided.

Honours year A compulsory BSc has been built into the new course, which is normally undertaken in year 4 or 5. The BSc is a modular degree programme and there are a wide range of subject choices, for example genetics,

Imperial

psychology, biochemistry and management (taught at the Imperial College Management School alongside MBA students). Some modules are taken in years 2 or 3.

Elective study/SSMs   There is a 12 week elective in year 6 (8 week study and 4 week holiday). SSMs in the final year cover four 2 week courses in subjects of your choice. There is a wide range of specialties to choose from.

Course details

Course length	● 6 years (5 for appropriately qualified graduates)
Total number of medical undergraduates	● c. 2000
Male/Female ratio	● 44:56

Admission procedure

Average A level requirements	● Under review but it was ABB (Chemistry plus at least one other Science or Maths)
Average Scottish Higher requirements	● Good grades at CSYS (ask admissions for advice on subjects)
Number of applicants (Sept 2000 entry)	● 2747
Proportion of applicants interviewed	● n/a
Make up of interview panel	● Chair, external clinician, academic, and clinical student
Months interviews held	● November–March
Number admitted (Sept 2000 entry)	● 326
Proposed entry size for 2001	● 326 to increase to 380 in 2002
Proportion of overseas students	● 7.4%
Proportion of mature students	● 5–10%
Faculty's view of taking a gap year	● Encouraged for students using the year constructively
Proportion taking Intercalated Hons	● Intercalated degree buit in to the course
Possibility of direct entrance to clinical phase	● Oxbridge only

Finances

Tuition fees per year	● £1050
Fees for self-funding students	● £1050
Fees for graduates	● £1050
Fees for overseas students	● £11 500 p.a. (pre-clinical) and £19 150 p.a. (clinical)
Assistance for elective funding	● 3 scholarships from 3 trusts
Assistance for travel to attachments	● None from University
Access and hardship funds	● Yes (students in final years tend to be more successful)

Average cost of living

Weekly rent	● Halls £58–£82 Private £70–£100
Pint of lager	● Union Bar £1.50 City Centre pub £2.30
Cinema	● £3.50–£8
Nightclub	● Free–£20

Course organisation The course being quite new and at a newly merged school, initially presented some problems. However, everyone has been keen to make Imperial a success and there is a genuine willingness to adapt and improve components of the course. The course runs well and most students believe it is successful and enjoyable.

PRHO year Almost all graduates stay in London, or the South East, as house officers in matching scheme posts.

The learning environment

The school uses a wide range of centres across central and west London for teaching. The main teaching hospitals – Charing Cross (in Hammersmith), Chelsea and Westminster (Fulham) and St Mary's (Paddington) – are supplemented by peripheral DGHs and teaching hospitals in Middlesex and Surrey. A new building (The Sir Alexander Fleming building) at the main Imperial College site is used for basic biomedical sciences. There are adequate public transport links between all sites and a new London Transport discount scheme has reduced some of the travel costs.

Library facilities There are libraries at all sites, which open late (7 p.m. or 12 a.m. for late night revision) on weekdays and are also open on Saturday mornings.

Computer facilities There is a considerable emphasis on IT in the Imperial course. To sustain this, the number of computer facilities is expanding considerably and training is also provided. There are computer facilities for Imperial College medical students at all peripheral attachments.

Clinical skills laboratory These are at Charing Cross and St Mary's hospitals. Students are encouraged to use them as part of their training in both timetabled and student arranged sessions. They are very well equipped and good fun to use.

Teaching hospitals The major sites are Charing Cross, Chelsea and Westminster and St Mary's hospitals. Other peripheral hospitals are also used. Teaching is generally better the smaller the group, and patients in the main teaching hospitals are sometimes prone to suffer "student fatigue" and may be disinclined to talk to students. This is not a problem at the peripheral sites. Hospital teaching is consultant led. There is sometimes little sense of belonging to a particular firm, because of frequently moving hospitals. This can undermine the clinical experience.

Student friendliness and support Students from the original medical schools integrated well and any pre-existing rivalry between St Mary's and Charing Cross has all but disappeared. There are very few students left who started out at the pre-merged schools. Students in earlier years, who are based at South Kensington, can feel remote from the medical environment. Soon after starting at Imperial, freshers are allocated a "parent" student from the year above. "Parents" are able to help you adjust to University and mecial school life. They also help you to ease in to the social life and can offer advice and tips about course work. Each student has a tutor who should be available for personal and academic problems and advice. Imperial College has counselling and welfare services.

Student life

The medical school has made a name for itself by incorporating the best of both its parent schools. The central London setting (on neutral Imperial College ground) and the wide range of people (10% graduate and 10% overseas) has assisted this process. Opportunities for non-medical pursuits abound but the traditional medical student lifestyle is in no danger of disappearing.

Imperial

Accommodation   First years have a guaranteed place in halls at about £70 per week. Halls are 2–30 minutes from one of the three main hospitals, and no more than an hour from all the peripheral sites. Private sector accommodation is expensive if you want to live near to Imperial College in central London (£75–£95+ per week).

Entertainment and societies   The Medical School's own Students Union and societies help Imperial medics maintain a separate identity from the rest of Imperial College students. However, medical students can also take advantage of Imperial College Union and its teams and clubs. There are student bars at both St Mary's and Charing Cross hospitals. Facilities at the Reynolds Building (Charing Cross) are due to undergo major refurbishment. Highlights of the year include Freshers Roadshow (Freshers week), the interyear rugby match, Rag week and the Summer Ball. There are plenty of medical student events spread through each term.

Sports facilities   Imperial College Medical School teams have grounds at Teddington and Cobham, and Imperial College has pitches and an astroturf at Gunnersbury. Students can also use three sports centres and local council pitches in the vicinity of the Medical School. The Imperial Medics Rugby team has already made itself a name at a European level and the school frequently holds many United Hospitals trophies.

The five BEST things about Imperial Medical School

- The Medical School has a great team spirit, with many excellent societies and clubs.

- You can choose between the close-knit medical community at the Medical School, the larger Imperial College environment or metropolitan city life.

- The ethos and tradition of the constituent medical schools combining in a new medical school makes it a vibrant and exciting time for Imperial students.

- A brand new building for biomedical sciences, at the South Kensington Imperial College site, as well as Chelsea and Westminster Hospital (known as the "Hilton Hospital") mean salubrious surroundings.

- Large city with a huge range of cultural activities – anything you want can be found.

The five WORST things about Imperial Medical School

- The new course has only recently been created and is still evolving so there may be limited advice from the older years. The course is likely to continue to evolve in the near future.

- Travel between sites adds to the expense of studying and can add stress.

- Split teaching hospital sites divides the year groups up.

- Imperial College is sometimes pictured as boring and academic.

- Expensive, polluted, over-populated, time-consuming dirty old London, etc.

Further information

Admissions: School of Medicine
Imperial College
LONDON
SW7 2AZ
Tel: 020 7589 5111
Fax: 020 7594 8004

1650 students
www: http://www.ucl.ac.uk

Royal Free and University College Medical School

One of the largest medical schools in the UK lies in an exciting, attractive and vibrant part of London. The Royal Free and University College London Medical School (RUMS) is the product of the recent merger of two world class institutions: Royal Free Hospital School of Medicine and University College London Medical School. Our parent college University College London (UCL) has an excellent reputation for teaching and research and RUMS offers a modern course, taught by respected academics and clinicians, alongside some very friendly students.

The course

Teaching and assessment   Starting in 2000 the new curriculum is a six year integrated systems-based course, including an intercalated BSc for non-graduates. This may be taken after years 2, 3, or 4. Clinical experience starts from day 1 although pre-clinical/clinical divide has not entirely been abandoned.

The core curriculum is arranged into three distinct phases.

Phase One: In phase one (Science and Medicine, years 1 and 2) the core curriculum consists of sequential systems-based modules including:

Year 1: Foundations of Health and Disease; Infection and Defence; Circulation and Breathing; Fluids, Nutrition and Metabolism; Cancer Biology.

Year 2: Movement and Musculoskeletal Biology; Neuroscience and Behaviour; Endocrine Systems; Reproduction, Genetics and Growth.

Phase Two: In Phase Two of the course (Science and Medical Practice, years 3 and 4) the core curriculum consists of a series of sequential clinical attachments, reflecting and building on the systems-based modules of Phase One. In year 3 there are two half days of formal teaching (including basic science) each week. In year 4 there are blocks of formal teaching (again including basic science) between clinical attachments.

151

Phase Three: In Phase Three of the course (Professional Development, year five) there are clinical attachments in general practice, accident and emergency and district general hospitals, as well as selective specialist clinical attachments and a period of elective study. This is followed by further experience at DGHs, a revision course, a period shadowing the house officer post you will be appointed to, and intensive revision of clinical skills.

Course details

Course length	● 6 years
Total number of medical undergraduates	● 1733
Male/Female ratio	● 50:50

Admission procedure

Average A level requirements	● AAB (Must include Chemistry)
Average Scottish Higher requirements	● Please check with the School
Number of applicants (Sept 2000 entry)	● 3000
Proportion of applicants interviewed	● 30%
Make up of interview panel	● Academic staff and a clinical student
Months interviews held	● November–March
Number admitted (Sept 2000 entry)	● 330
Proposed entry size for 2001	● 330
Proportion of overseas students	● 7%
Proportion of mature students	● 15%
Faculty's view of taking a gap year	● Positive
Proportion taking Intercalated Hons	● Compulsory
Possibility of direct entrance to clinical phase	● Oxbridge only

Finances

Tuition fees per year	● £1050
Fees for self-funding students	● £1050
Fees for graduates	● £1050
Fees for overseas students	● £12 475
Assistance for elective funding	● Yes
Assistance for travel to attachments	● Yes
Access and hardship funds	● Students may apply but must already have taken a loan

Average cost of living

Weekly rent	● Halls £45–£100 Private £60–£100
Pint of lager	● Union Bar £1.40 City Centre pub £2.20
Cinema	● £3.50–£10
Nightclub	● Free–£20

Running throughout these sequential modules for all five years of the course there are three vertical modules: Mechanisms of Drug Action/Use of Medicines; Society and the Individual; and Pathology. There is also a continuous strand of Professional Development from year 1 through to year 5.

Special Study Modules   In addition to the core curriculum there are special study modules to permit study of selected aspects in depth. These may be medical or non-medical and can include law, history of medicine, arts and modern language. Four must be taken in Phase One, three in Phase Two and two in Phase Three.

Assessment   Assessment is integrated, with a considerable amount of formative assessment and a portfolio of course work that must be completed to a satisfactory standard in order to permit entry to end of year summative assessments which determine progression. Assessment includes MCQS, OSCEs and oral examinations.

Placements outside the university   Most clinical teaching will be in the UCL/Middlesex, Royal Free and Whittington hospitals, all of which are within central London. District general hospital attachments are normally in outer London (Barnet, Northwick Park, Stanmore, North Middlesex), or further afield (for example King's Lynn and Northampton).

Honours year   An intercalated degree is compulsory for all non-graduate students on the course. There is a very wide range of subjects on offer, many arts or non-medically based.

Elective study   A period of elective study is taken in the final year. Most students choose to spend this abroad. Limited funding may be available.

Course organisation   Student feedback on course quality and teaching is actively sought through questionnaires, faculty education committees and staff-student consultative committees. Courses will be changed in the light of (valid) student comments. Organisation is generally very good with comprehensive lecture notes provided by most lecturers. Lectures and formal tutorials still form an important part of the new course.

PRHO year   At present, the old medical schools each run a matching scheme featuring jobs in central and greater London. However, competition for the teaching hospital is extremely high.

The learning environment

Most teaching in Phase One is based on the main Gower St Campus of UCL, making particular use of the Cruciform and Rockefeller Buildings. These have recently been refurbished and have two lecture theatres equipped with audio-visual and computer presentation facilities, three wet laboratories, two dry laboratories and a modern topographical anatomy laboratory/dissection room, as well as a clinical skills laboratory and a suite of seminar rooms.

Library facilities   There are large medical and clinical science libraries on the Gower St Campus, a well-stocked and spacious library on the Royal Free Campus, and a new and well-stocked library on the Archway (Whittington Hospital) campus. In addition, the many post-graduate medical institutes associated with UCL have specialist libraries within easy walking distance of the Gower St Campus.

Computer facilities   There are clusters of networked computers throughout all RUMS campus sites and many halls of residence. When they are not booked for formal teaching, students have free access, on a first-come first-served basis. Most networked computers are Windows pcs, although there are some clusters of Apple computers. All students have free internet and email access, as well as a wide variety of networked software. IT skills are assessed at the beginning of the course, and there is a scheme for peer-tutoring.

Clinical skills laboratories   There are clinical skills laboratories on all three "home" campuses, and in addition to timetabled sessions, students may arrange access at other times. They are all well liked by students allowing such diverse activities as suturing sponges, canulating plastic arms and catheterising large plastic penises.

Teaching hospitals   In Phase One students spend one day each week on one of the three clinical campuses (The Royal Free Hospital, UCL/Middlesex Hospital and the Whittington Hospital) or in the community. In year 3 clinical attachments are mainly at these "home" campuses, or in general practice. In years 4 and 5 a variety of DGHs are also used (see above). A new skyscraping UCH is due to open in c. 2005 to replace the current UCH and Middlesex Hospital.

Student friendliness and support   In Phase One all students are assigned to a personal tutor/academic adviser who is a normally a basic scientist, and who will oversee their personal and academic development and provide pastoral care. In Phases Two and Three students are assigned to personal tutors who are clinically qualified. In addition, the faculty tutorial team provide regular "walk-in surgeries", and most academic staff in UCL have an open-door policy or clearly advertised hours when they are available to students. UCL has a wide range of welfare, support and counselling services available for students.

Student life

From the day you arrive at RUMS you will become part of a large but close knit family that will ensure your days here are comfortable and enjoyable. You will be assigned a "parent" of the opposite sex from whom you should attempt to glean notes, books and drinks at all opportunities. They will tell you what to go to and what to avoid!

Medical students have their own bar/clubhouse in Huntley St on the Gower St Campus, as well as social and union facilities at the Royal Free Campus. In addition, there is the main UCL Union, with centres on the Gower St Campus and in the Windeyer Building (part of the Middlesex Hospital site a few minutes walk from Gower St). The University of London Union (ULU) is a stone's throw from the Gower St Campus. This means there is an unparalleled variety of sports and social facilities available, with opportunities to remain within a (mainly) medical environment, or to meet students from other disciplines.

Accommodation   Nearly 100% of 1st year students stay in UCL or University of London halls. Halls are generally acceptable and a second year in halls is normally available during the BSc or final year. The accommodation office at Senate House offers help and legal advice to London students. To find better value accommodation, many students choose to travel into central London from places like Finsbury Park and Camden.

Entertainment and societies   At RUMS we live up to the medical student reputation in style. Your motto will become "work hard, play hard" and you will soon learn to recognise the underside of every table in the medic bars! The well loved events you see year after year draw the whole crowd. The awesome atmosphere created at the "big nights" is down to two things: everyone knows everyone else, and everyone is having a great time. We offer theme nights, barbecues, comedy, live music and a host of other memorable one-offs. We run three balls a year where everyone dresses up and parties 'til late to live music in glamorous surroundings with fairground rides in the background! There is always something going on...

One of the most anticipated events is Rag week, which is an orgy of money collecting for charity. You'll get up at 5 a.m. to shake a tin at a tube station and go to bed at 3 a.m. having exhausted yourself at a party or pub-crawl. These weeks are a massive event in the social calendar that we all look forward to.

We run our own sports clubs, which play all over London and further afield (see below). The team spirit in these clubs is tremendous. They organise social events ranging from "civilised" dinners to rather less civilised initiations. Our societies put on plays and musical shows alongside gigs and choral performances. The infamous revues, drawn from the tradition of both old schools, are high points of the year with everyone turning out to watch friends make idiots of themselves.

At RUMS you are not confined to socialising within the medical school – you also have the varied clubs and societies of UCL to explore.

Sports facilities   RUMS and ULU have sports fields all over London with the main medics' field up in Enfield (north London). There are swimming pools in John Astor House – free for medics – and at ULU. We have use of the ULU boathouses for rowing.

The five BEST things about RUMS

- Friendly atmosphere and close medical community within a larger college.

- Central London location within walking distance of some of the finest theatres, concert halls and museums in the world, as well as being in the centre of historic Bloomsbury. The Royal Free Campus has both the cosmopolitan atmosphere of Hampstead and the open country of Hampstead Heath.

- Plenty of opportunity to mix with non-medics at a multi-faculty university.

- A major centre of biomedical research, with opportunities to work alongside world leaders in research.

- RUMS medics are members of their own Union, the UCL Union and the University of London Union so there is no shortage of student activity.

The five WORST things about RUMS

- Central London location, with main roads between many buildings. It's very busy!

- Need to travel outside London for playing fields and between Gower St (UCH), Archway (Whittington) and Hampstead (Royal Free) on the Northern line.

- Living in London is bl**dy expensive. Don't underestimate this!

- In a class of 330 it can be easy to be isolated and not meet all of your fellow students, especially in the early years.

- Being so close to the Strand Polytechnic (aka King's).

Further information

Admissions: Dr B Cross,
Faculty Tutor,
Faculty of Life Sciences,
UCL,
London WC1E 6BT,
Tel: 020 7209 6321, email: n.quinn@ucl.ac.uk
www.ucl.ac.uk/medical school

Students Union: Brian Hogan,
Medical Students' & Sites' Officer,
25 Gordon Street,
London, WC1H 0AY
Tel: 020 7679 7949, email: mss.officer@ucl.ac.uk
www.uclu.org.uk

1200 students
Email: admissions@qmw.ac.uk
www: http://www.mds.qmw.ac.uk

St Bartholomew's and the Royal London School of Medicine and Dentistry (at Queen Mary and Westfield College)

The Medical School of St Bartholomew's and the Royal London is situated in the City of London and the East End, home to stockbrokers, Jack the Ripper and the Krays. The East End is also home to a young, vibrant, but poverty stricken multicultural community in great need of decent healthcare and with fascinating pathology. To cater for their needs, a new multi-million pound hospital is being built on the Royal London site in Whitechapel. The future of Bart's hospital is now secure as a specialist centre for disciplines including cancer, cardiothoracic surgery, urology and endocrinology.

The new school is the largest faculty of Queen Mary and Westfield, which, in turn, is part of the University of London. The school, based on the oldest medical school at the Royal London and the oldest hospital, 900 year old Barts, was the first London medical school to complete the merger process, so most of the problems associated with this have been ironed out.

The course

Students starting after 2000 are following a new curriculum centred on problem-based learning. There are only a few lectures and students have to find their own answers to clinical problems using textbooks, journals and the internet. All students follow the same core course, but more emphasis is now placed on individually selected Special Study Modules (SSMs). The traditional pre-clinical/clinical division has gone as the new course integrates basic medical, human, and clinical sciences from day 1 until graduation. A welcome change is that students are sent on GP placements and to hospital clinics from the first year.

Dissection is no longer part of the core course, and anatomy is taught using computer-aided learning programmes, anatomical models and prosected (already dissected) specimens. Those who wish to dissect may do this as a SSM.

157

Teaching and assessment   Teaching is systems based, concentrating on health for the first part of the course and disease for the second. Instead of studying anatomy, physiology, and pharmacology separately, all aspects of a body system, such as the cardiovascular system, will be considered as an integrated whole. Excellent and well-established courses in communication skills (using actors and videotaping) and ethics run as threads throughout the 5 years.

Course details

Course length	● 5 years
Total number of medical undergraduates	● 1200
Male/Female ratio	● 50:50

Admission procedure

Average A level requirements	● AAB Chemistry plus one other Science
Average Scottish Higher requirements	● AAAAB with CSYS in either Chemistry or Biology at grade B
Number of applicants (Sept 2000 entry)	● 1720
Number of applicants interviewed	● 940
Make up of interview panel	● Clinician, Basic medical scientist, and clinical student
Months interviews held	● October–March
Number admitted (Sept 2000 entry)	● 241
Proposed entry size for 2001	● n/a
Proportion of overseas students	● 8%
Proportion of mature students	● 5–10%
Faculty's view of taking a gap year	● Very supportive if applicants have positive plans for the year
Proportion taking Intercalated Hons	● 50%
Possibility of direct entrance to clinical phase	● Yes, for Oxbridge students

Finances

Tuition fees per year	● £1050
Fees for self-funding students	● £1050
Fees for graduates	● £1050
Fees for overseas students	● £10 150 p.a. (pre-clinical) and £18 000 p.a. (clinical)
Assistance for elective funding	● Some
Assistance for travel to attachments	● No
Access and hardship funds	● College administers Access-type funds

Average cost of living

Weekly rent	● Halls £60–£100 Private £50+ (average £70)
Pint of lager	● Union Bar £1.50 City Centre pub £1.50–£2
Cinema	● £2.50+
Nightclub	● £3+

Summer exams are set for years 1–4 of the course, but there will be no "big bang" final examinations as in the past. Examiners use negatively marked multiple-choice and extended matching questions for nearly all subjects, and short- and long-answer questions seem to be disappearing. Marks for problem-based learning count for up to 50% of the final grade. At the end of the 5th year students are assessed on their "competence to practise" as a PRHO and must pass an integrated paper and clinical exams.

Placements outside the university   Students can expect to be sent to attachments outside the main teaching hospitals. Placements are in district generals and other associated hospitals (accommodation free). Destinations include seaside Southend and the semi-military hospital at Frimley Park. GP attachments and SSMs can be arranged country-wide.

Honours year   Both BSc and BMedSci courses are offered. Popular courses include neuroanatomy and the Bachelor of Medical Science (BMedSci), but some students have studied anthropology, psychology and even German, although this kind of choice is rare. Students can choose to stay at QM or go to another college for this year. Fees are payable for the year but some funding is available.

Elective study/SSMs   The elective lasts 2–3 months, starting after Christmas in the 5th year of the course. There are some existing arrangements with institutions world wide, which can make for easier organisation of the trip. Students can go almost anywhere as long as they can find themselves a supervisor. SSMs and some 3–month attachments can be spent at partner institutions in Europe. Other 1 month modules can be chosen from a variety of subjects: clinical, research, complementary medicine, journalism. The number and variety of SSMs will increase with the introduction of the new course. The ERASMUS project offers 3-month exchange placements anywhere in Europe.

Course organisation   At present the course is very well organised: schedules are available well in advance and learning objectives are clearly stated for every course. Students get tons of pre-printed lecture notes, and there is an opportunity to appraise all lectures and lecturers. Students are listened to and changes happen because of the active staff/student committee and the curriculum committee.

PRHO year   There are sufficient posts in the South East and London for all graduates. Posts are allocated through a matching scheme of applications with students and consultants, each putting down their choices in rank order and a computer working out how to create the greatest happiness for the greatest number. Some people go for jobs "off-scheme", i.e. in hospitals associated with other medical schools, all over the country. The new curriculum emphasises that the PRHO year will be regarded as an extension of the course and will provide continuing education and personal supervision.

The learning environment

The three sites (Bart's, the London, and QM) are all within 3 miles of each other in the City and East End of London. They are easily accessible by tube and bicycle. The basic medical sciences (BMS) department at QM, Mile End where lower years are based, has excellent high-tech facilities and teaching. Bar Med is a cafe bar attached to the (BMS) building where students escape for coffee between lectures. Many of the district general hospitals used are in or close to the East End and accessible by bike, bus or tube.

Library facilities   There are three large libraries, one at each site. The two hospital libraries have wonderful architecture, history, and atmosphere. QM is large and spacious but tends to be very noisy during the daytime. Libraries are open 9 a.m.–9 p.m. on weekdays, 9 a.m.–4 p.m. on Saturdays. The QM library is also open on Sundays from 1 p.m.–7 p.m. There are two large pathology museums at the hospitals, which include the Elephant Man's skeleton among the exhibits. The pathology museum at the London is accessible 24 hours a day. Libraries include computers, Medline search facilities, and videos.

Computer facilities   The school is well equipped on all three sites. All computing facilities and functions are available and regularly updated. Computers are increasingly used for teaching. Computers are available during library hours and from 10 a.m.-8 p.m. at weekends. The computer rooms at Barts and QM are open late. There are also computer facilities at South Woodford halls.

Clinical skills laboratory   Barts was the first medical college to establish a clinical skills lab for use by medics and nurses. The clinical skills centre is available to everyone in the school. First years learn clinical skills in an adapted ward at Mile End hospital.

Teaching hospitals   St Bartholomew's and the Royal London Hospitals are the home sites for teaching. Barts is historic, beautiful and very specialist. It no longer has an accident and emergency department, so it is very calm compared to the London. The Royal London Hospital provides both general and specialist services to the local community, so students see a wide range of common conditions, as well as specialist trauma cases brought in by the Helicopter Emergency Medical Service (HEMS).

Student friendliness and support   On the first day of college, freshers are assigned a senior student to act as their "parent" and guide them through the first few weeks and beyond. Student parents introduce their "children" to their friends, take them out to dinner and offer advice on all issues, from simple things such as work to more complicated matters such as your love life. This makes for a lot of integration between students from different years. All students are allocated their own academic tutor; for personal and other problems they have use of a pastoral pool of sympathetic doctors and senior lecturers. The Medical and Dental Students Association appoints a student as Welfare Officer, as does QM college. Counselling is available within 24 hours at QM college. Those with mental health problems can be seen in confidence by a consultant at another teaching hospital in a reciprocal arrangement with the school.

Student life

Student social life revolves around the Association/Union buildings at both Barts and the London. The Medical Student President is head of the Medical and Dental Students Association and takes a paid year out from his or her studies solely to represent and protect the interests of the medical and dental student community. The soon to be refurbished Association building at the London and the bar at Barts are for use by medics, dentists and their guests. There is a café-bar and bookshop in the Clubs Union building at the London. The official Association magazine, M.A.D., comes out at least twice a term and reports on social, sporting and other events.

Accommodation   Students choose whether they wish to live in Queen Mary College or University of London (intercollegiate) accommodation and whether they wish to be catered for or cook for themselves. QM halls include former medical college residences at Barts and at the London; these are mostly occupied by medics.

Most senior students would advise freshers to apply for accommodation at Floyer House, Whitechapel or College Hall at Barts. South Woodford halls of residence are the cheapest option but a 20-minutes tube ride away. In central London students from all colleges of the University of London live together in intercollegiate halls. These are also a 20 minute tube ride away from college. With all residences students should check whether or not rent is payable during holidays. The tube pass to South Woodford or central London costs approximately £45 per month with a student discount card.

Most senior students live in the East End in shared houses. Almost everyone lives within walking distance of the Royal London and QM sites. Property is slightly cheaper in East London compared to other parts of the capital. The Griffin Community Trust provides cheap (approx £50 per week), luxurious housing in a very special development incorporating housing for the elderly, a community centre and flats for clinical students. Student residents spend an hour or two a week with their elderly neighbours and play bingo, watch videos or just chat. Both students and elders say how much they gain from the experience.

Entertainment and societies   The Medical and Dental Students Association is thriving and provides social and sporting opportunities and welfare services for all. The two medical student bars at Barts and The London hold regular discos and theme nights. Wednesdays (after sports matches) and Fridays are the big nights for going out. The summer ball at Barts rivals that of any Oxbridge college, and there are smaller balls for freshers' week, Rag and at Christmas. The Burns' Night supper is very popular, incorporating kilt wearing and ceilidh dancing. There are Rag and freshers' events every night during their respective weeks. Rag week is huge and students raked in over £150 000 last year from street collections, marathon running, bed pushing and a fashion show. A large TV screen in the bar regularly shows the main sports events.

There are over 30 clubs and societies run by the association offer the chance to develop new interests, meet people, place sport and have a good time. Amongst the most active societies are: the drama society, which stages productions every term, including the infamous Christmas show; the Asian Society; the Music Society, which includes the choir, orchestra, brass groups, and several bands; and the religious societies. The Art and Photography Club has its own art room and a dark room at the London.

Sports facilities   The Association clubs cater for nearly all sporting interests and most welcome beginners. There are two off-site sports grounds, swimming pools at both Barts and the London, gyms at Barts, QM college and South Woodford halls, squash at Barts and QM, tennis and badminton courts. There is rowing locally on the River Lea and on the Thames. Hockey, water polo, women's football and rugby have had good successes in recent years.

The five BEST things about Barts and the London Medical School

- A brand new course, innovative curriculum and teaching.

- All students and visitors agree that we are a very friendly community with a close-knit, old medical school atmosphere. Students tend to have friends from all years rather than just their own.

- Reasonable rents for shared houses, considering that we are in the centre of London and everyone lives close to each other.

- There are good year-round events, and Bart's bar opens with regular late licences. The local area is getting very trendy with new bars and restaurants opening all the time.

- Diverse area, with a wide range of things to do and cultures to experience.

The five WORST things about Barts and the London Medical School

- Local areas – we are surrounded by very deprived communities, and, whilst this means good clinical experience and pathology subject matter, it can be a bit depressing.

- Travelling – there is some travelling between sites required, and the rush hour lasts for hours.

- Little interaction with non-medical students, and some bad feeling between the medics and QM students. However, this is improving.

- London is such a massive place that it can take you some time to feel at ease with its vastness.

- Expense – living and studying in London is more expensive than elsewhere.

Further information

Admissions: Admissions Office
Queen Mary College
Turner Street
London
E1 2AD
Fax: 020 7377 7612
Tel: 020 7377 7611

St George's

St George's Hospital Medical School (SGHMS) is located in the heart of Tooting, in south London. It is a very welcoming school, with plenty of atmosphere and plenty of patients for budding doctors to fulfil all their needs without ever having to look elsewhere. St George's Hospital itself is one of the largest teaching hospitals in the UK, situated in a heavily populated part of London with pressing health needs. As well as medics, there are nursing, midwifery, physiotherapy, radiography and biomedical science students at St George's, all of whom mix well with staff to create a strong feeling of community within the hospital. It is this, in particular, which makes SGHMS a great place to study. Most will thoroughly enjoy the atmosphere, but all will, at the very least, appreciate it.

St George's

Stop press

St George's also offers a new four year fast-track medical degree course to graduate entrants. The first intake of 35 began their studies in September 2000.

Where possible we have given details for the graduate entry programme:

Course length	● 4 years
Total number of places	● 70 (2001 entry)
Admission requirements	● see below
Admission process	● Written test (GAMSAT) followed, for those doing well in the test, by a selection day including structured interviews.
Number of applicants	● 360 (2000 entry)
Proportion of applicants reaching interview stage	● n/a
Tuition fees per year	● £1050 (first year only)

Further information: http:www.sghms.ac.uk/agep

The course

The course lasts 5 years, with clinical experience starting with visits to GP surgeries in the first year. Since 1996 all new medical students have undertaken the new Special Study Modules (SSMs) at St George's. The aim of the SSM programme is to allow students to study, in depth, areas of particular interest to them.

Course details

Course length	● 5 years
Total number of medical undergraduates	● c. 1000
Male/Female ratio	● 52:48

Admission procedure

Average A level requirements	● ABB – must include Chemistry
Average Scottish Higher requirements	● ABB at CSYS
Number of applicants (Sept 2000 entry)	● c. 1800
Proportion of applicants interviewed	● 25%
Make up of interview panel	● 3 academic staff
Months interviews held	● November–March
Number admitted (Sept 2000 entry)	● 187
Proposed entry size for 2001	● 187
Proportion of overseas students	● 7%
Proportion of mature students	● 5%
Faculty's view of taking a gap year	● Acceptable
Proportion taking Intercalated Hons	● 30%
Possibility of direct entrance to clinical phase	● Oxbridge applicants only

Finances

Tuition fees per year	● £1050
Fees for self-funding students	● £1050
Fees for graduates	● £1050
Fees for overseas students	● £9085 p.a. (pre-clinical) and £16 225 p.a. (clinical)
Assistance for elective funding	● Yes
Assistance for travel to attachments	● Yes fully reimbursed
Access and hardship funds	● Yes

Average cost of living

Weekly rent	● Halls £45 Private £60
Pint of lager	● Union Bar £1.25 City Centre pub £1.90
Cinema	● £2–£7
Nightclub	● Free–£20 (easy access to London's West End)

Teaching and assessment   In the first year there is a foundation module in the first term. Then the rest of the teaching is divided into two core cycles: cycles 1 and 2. In core cycle 1 (years 1 and 2), students study systems modules integrated with some clinical experience and undertake two SSMs. In core cycle 2 (years 3–5) students get general clinical experience in hospitals, GP surgeries etc., along with some speciality clinical teaching and two more SSMs. Exams take place every term through years 1–4 and all contribute to the final MBBS qualification. The fifth year is exam free apart from finals in June!

Assessment takes the form of written exams: MCQs (sounds easy but they're negatively marked), short answer questions and the odd essay, and synoptic assessments.

Placements outside the university   From the third year, students are placed at a variety of different other hospitals for speciality training. Much training will take place at St George's. There is a usually a choice of where you go, travel expenses are reimbursed and accommodation is free.

Honours year   An intercalated BSc can be taken after the second, third or fourth year. The later the degree is taken the more clinical in nature it can be. Study can be at St George's Hospital or other London colleges/medical schools (or further afield if you so desire) with a wide range of courses available – choices are not restricted to medical or science subjects.

Elective study/SSMs   The elective is taken in the fifth year. It can be done almost anywhere in the world with the only limit being your imagination. It lasts for 2 months and help with funding is sometimes available.

Course organisation   The course is well organised, with easy access to members of staff and administration officers if any queries arise about aspects of the course. There is an education officer elected from the student body) who helps with staff/student liaisons and course organisation. Students in other years are usually willing to help with any work problems, give you advice or sell you their old books.

PRHO year   St George's operates a matching scheme for its students to get house officer posts in those hospitals it is affiliated to. Most students are usually offered a place from this scheme, and the option is open for students to arrange their own PRHO job.

The learning environment

The Medical School is part of the main teaching hospital, but it occupies a distinct area of the hospital itself. There are six floors containing the library, computer rooms, teaching theatres, clinical labs, offices and student area. The main hospital including shop and canteen is easily accessed from the Medical School. On the second floor is the School Club (equivalent of a students union), consisting of a bar, student offices, a coffee shop, school bookshop, games room, music room and snooker room. Many students and staff go there to relax for lunch and coffee breaks, and many of the extracurricular activities are held there. There is also a student shop downstairs.

Library facilities   These are extensive, with about 40 000 books, 800 journals on current subscription, and a total of 77 000 journals available. Other facilities include inter-library loans, photocopying, a large history and archive collection, and an audio-visual room with a large variety of video material (seven video players).

Computer facilities   An excellent range of computing facilities are available with networked database, CD-ROM and interactive media. The library has a Unicorn catalogue for public access, 100 workstations for network access, 11 workstations for Word for Windows, one Excel workstation and scanner facilities. There is also a large 24 hour access computer room in the Medical School (Windows and multi-media) with about 30 terminals. A computer room with eight computer stations is at the halls of residence.

Clinical skills laboratories   These are large and well equipped with TV monitors and audio systems for large-group teaching. Numerous cubicles are located around the Medical School for individual and group teaching of clinical skills.

Teaching hospitals   In addition to the time spent at St George's, students will be able to study at a wide variety of DGHs in quite near proximity to Tooting. The main ones are St Helier's Hospital in Sutton, and Atkinson Morley Hospital (neurology) in Wimbledon.

Student friendliness and support   Students at George's believe they are renowned far and wide for their friendliness and easy-going nature. Whether this is true is debatable but there is a strong school spirit and students are supportive of each other. All freshers are assigned a "Mother" or "Father" student to look after them in their first year. There is normally no problem in borrowing lecture notes and getting useful advice. George's students are always ready to help a friend. The school has counselling services locally, and students can use ULU (University of London Union) facilities.

Student life

First and foremost, St George's is now the only free-standing medical school in the UK. The only other students around the place are in the caring professions or professions allied to medicine. There is a great feeling of camaraderie in the college – you will get to know most people in your year and many others. There is much mixing between year groups and with students of the other disciplines. This is partly because there are so many social events organised by the Student Union. The Medical School itself encourages students and staff to take as positive an attitude to their extracurricular interests as it does to studying.

Accommodation   In their first year students can live in halls, which, at only 15 minutes walking distance from the school and costing only £45 per week, may be one of the best deals in London! There is a downside – rooms in halls are a bit on the small side, and baths, toilets and kitchen facilities may have to be shared between six to eight people. Tooting itself is filled with eager landlords waiting to accommodate local medical students, and rents in the area are more favourable than in many other parts of London.

Entertainment and societies   St George's Bar is one of the biggest and cheapest bars in the country, and is the scene of many a great night for many medical students. Discos on alternate Friday nights, comedy nights and bands are well attended, and much fun is had by all. There is a wide screen TV with Satellite, and films and important football, rugby matches, etc. are regularly shown in the bar. The Cinema Club is very popular, showing films regularly in one of the large student auditoriums. It shows very recently released films, some pre-video releases, and, of course, popcorn is provided!

There is a colossal range of societies and clubs to join, from all the conventional sporting ones like rugby and cricket to a parachuting club and a hill walking society. There are various religious societies, the orchestra and musical societies, also a debating society – the list is endless. The school club is very supportive of new clubs, so if you come here and don't like any of the clubs you can set up your own!

Sports facilities   For the major outdoor sports, St George's uses its own sports ground at Cobham, which is located in a very rural part of south London (it is in Surrey actually). The rowing teams use the Boat House at Chiswick where many other London colleges row. At the hospital itself is the Rob Lowe Sports Centre which has six squash courts, two general fitness rooms with exercise bikes, treadmills, rowing machines, and step machines. There is also a weights room and a large sports hall for team sports like five-a-side football and basketball. There are regular circuit training and aerobic lessons.

The five BEST things about St George's Medical School

- The students – some of the best bunch of easy-going, fun-loving guys and girls you'll ever meet.

- The medical staff – some of the best bunch of easy-going, fun-loving guys and girls you'll ever meet.

- The location – in south London, away from the main bustle of everyday life in central London, yet a stone's throw away from the heart of the most happening city in the world!

- The new fully integrated course – this has been designed to make medicine a much more clinically relevant and enjoyable.

- The bar – as the 8th wonder of the world, its ability to transform from serene area of rest where staff and students mingle at lunch and coffee breaks, to becoming something akin to a crime scene on some nights, is a modern miracle. Definitely the heart (and soul) of the Medical School.

The five WORST things about St George's Medical School

- Parking – if you've got a car, parking within a 2 mile radius of the hospital is like mission impossible.

- Canteen – over-priced, over-staffed and under-cooked. Your best bet is the great sandwiches they serve at the bar.

- Access to computers – with so many medical, nursing and postgraduate students at SGHMS, finding a free terminal in the library can sometimes be a problem in busy periods.

- Negatively marked MCQs (multiple choice questions) – many a great foot soldier has fallen at the last hurdle because of the excessive use of this weapon of mass destruction in exams!

- Although you are at a London medical school, St George's cannot pretend it is in central London.

Further information

British Medical Association

The British Medical Association (BMA) is both the doctor's professional organisation and trade union protecting the professional and personal interests of its members. It is the voice of the medical profession in the UK and represents the profession internationally. Members and staff are in constant touch with ministers, government departments, members of parliament and other influential bodies – conveying to them the profession's views on healthcare and health policy. Over 80% of practising doctors and the majority of medical students are members. The BMA's head office is based in London, but there are three offices in Scotland, one each in Northern Ireland and Wales and 13 regional offices in England. The BMA is a medical publisher in its own right but also includes the BMJ Publishing Group. The BMJ Publishing Group is a major medical and scientific publisher and publishes the weekly *British Medical Journal* and the monthly *Student BMJ*.

The Medical Students Committee represents students within the Association and also to important outside bodies, such as the Departments of Education and Health and the General Medical Council. Through the committee the BMA campaigns on many issues, such as student finances and debt, reforms of the medical degree syllabus, and health and safety. Following devolution the BMA has established MSCs in Northern Ireland, Scotland and Wales. There are student representatives of the BMA in every medical school and the BMA runs many local events and talks for students. Medical students who are members of the BMA receive a variety of benefits, including a free subscription to *Student BMJ,* free guidance notes, library and information services, and book discounts, to name but a few.

Medical Students Committee
British Medical Association
BMA House
Tavistock Square
London
WC1H 9JP

Tel: 020 7387 4499
Fax: 020 7383 6494
E-mail: iurmston@bma.org.uk
WWW: http://www.bma.org.uk

Becoming a doctor

General information on getting into medical schools is available from the BMA website.

Medical careers: a general guide (3rd revised edition): this publication is available free of charge to BMA members, from their local BMA office, or at £10 to non-members from the BMJ Bookshop. Tel: 020 7383 6244.

Student BMJ

The *Student BMJ is* an international journal specifically for medical students. It is published monthly and includes articles on education, medical careers, student life, science and news. Many of the articles and papers are written by medical students. Individuals or schools and libraries can subscribe to the journal.

For more information or a sample copy contact:

Student BMJ	Tel:	020 7383 6402
BMJ Publishing Group	Fax:	020 7383 6270
BMA House	Email:	bmjsubs@dial.pipex.com
Tavistock Square	www:	http://www.studentbmj.com
London WC1H WR		

Universities Central Admissions Service (UCAS)

Universities and Colleges Admissions Service	Tel:	01242 222444
Rose Hill	www:	http://www.ucas.com
New Barn Lane		
Cheltenham		
Gloucestershire		
GL52 3LZ		

- *UCAS Handbook and Application Form*   Essential reading and material for applicants to university courses.

- *Medical Courses 2000* £12.99.

National Union of Students (NUS)

National Union of Students	Tel:	020 7272 8900
Nelson Mandela House	Fax:	020 7263 5713
461 Holloway Road	Email:	nusuk@nus.org.uk
London		
N7 6LJ		

There are 15 information leaflets available from the NUS:

1–3	Student Awards (general information), Dependants' Allowances and Older Students' Allowance, Table of Rates for Awards and Allowances	9	Social Security Benefits
		10	Alternative Financial Assistance
		11	Postgraduate Awards
		12	Discretionary Awards – Appeals and Judicial Review
4	Means Testing of Mandatory Awards		
5	Student Loans	13	EU Students – Fees and Awards
6	Council Tax	14	Access Funds
7	National Insurance	15	Scottish Students – HE and FE
8	Income Tax		

Student Funding

Department for Education and Employment

Tel: 0800 731 9133
Email: info@dfee.gov.uk
www: http://www.open.gov.uk/dfee/support

The Scottish Office

www: http://www.scotland.gov.uk

There are many publications about higher education and funding for Scottish students available on the Web, or from:

The Stationery Office   Tel: 0131 228 4181
71 Lothian Road   Fax: 0131 622 7017
Edinburgh
EH3 9AZ

Charities

Copies of the following books should be available in the reference section of most public libraries:

- *The Charities Digest* – published by the Family Welfare Association

- *Money to Study* – published by UKOSA/NUS/EGAS

- *The Educational Grants Directory* – published by the Directory of Social Change

- *Directory of Grant-Making Trusts* – published by Charities Aid Foundation/Biblios

The British Medical Association Charities Office (see BMA address) has information about awards and grants for mature and second degree medical students.

Christian Medical Fellowship (CMF)

Dr Peter Saunders   Tel: 020 7928 4694
Student Secretary   Fax: 020 7620 2453
Christian Medical Fellowship Email: Student@cmf.org.uk or admin@cmf.org.uk
157 Waterloo Road   www: http://www.cmf.org.uk
London
SE1 8XN

CMF has over 5,500 medical student and doctor members throughout the UK and Ireland. It exists to encourage fellowship, Christian ethics, evangelism, medical mission, and to provide a Christian voice on medical issues. CMF runs conferences, co-ordinates local groups, and publishes widely at the interface of Christianity and medicine. It is one of 70 member bodies of the International Christian Medical and Dental Association (ICMDA).

A publications catalogue and information about local groups, conferences, and activities are available from the above address.

Medical Students International Network (MedSIN)

Founded in 1997, MedSIN is an independent, student-run organisation, which aims to facilitate medical students' involvement in humanitarian and educational activities at local, national, and international level. MedSIN groups in medical schools carry out sex education projects, international exchanges, bone marrow registration drives, seminars on topical issues and much more.

Through its membership of the International Federation of Medical Students' Association (IFMSA) MedSIN also provides opportunities to go on projects all over the world, from Angola to Zimbabwe. The IFMSA was founded in 1951 and promotes international co-operation on professional training and the achievement of humanitarian ideals.

To get in touch or find out more visit the MedSIN website: www.medsin.org

Gay and Lesbian Association of Doctors and Dentists(GLADD)

Email: gladd@dircon.co.uk   www: http://www.gladd.dircon.co.uk

GLADD was formed in 1995. It has an active student section and provides professional support, educational and social meetings both locally and nationally. GLADD campaigns vigorously within the health service and country at large on issues of equality relating to the lesbian, gay, and bisexual community.

Armed Forces: Cadet Recruitment

Royal Army Medical Corps: Tel: 01252 340307
Officer Recruiting   Fax: 01252 340224
Regimental Headquarters RAMC   Email: ramc.recruiting@army.mod.uk.net
Keogh Barracks
Ash Vale
Aldershot
Hants
GU12 5RQ

RAF:
Medical and Dental Liaison Officer
Directorate of Recruiting and Selection (Royal Air Force)
PO Box 1000
Cranwell
Sleaford
Lincolnshire
NG34 8GZ

Tel: 01400 261201 ext 6811
Fax 01400 262220
Email: mdlo@royalairforce.net

Royal Navy:
Med Pers (N)2
Room 133
Victory Building
HM Naval Base
Portsmouth
PO1 3LS

Tel: 02392 727818
Fax: 02392 727805

Further Reading

- *The New Learning* Medicine by Peter Richards (formerly Dean of St Mary's Medical School) and Simon Stockill, published by BMJ Publishing Group and updated regularly. Now in its 15th edition, this title is available from the BMJ Bookshop, Burton Street, London WC1H 9JR. Price £13.95 (discount available for BMA members). Tel: 020 7383 6185.

Glossary

Medicine is full of jargon and abbreviation. Estimates suggest students' vocabularies double over the course of a 5-year medical degree. Unfortunately, it is such a part of life for medical students and doctors that they sometimes forget to speak in plain language to the general public. The following is a very brief list of words pertaining to medical education that you are likely to come across in this guide, and perhaps in medical school prospectuses. Our apologies for any jargon we have used in the guide not listed here!

Anatomy: The study of the structure of the body. While this used to be taught by dissection, prosections (pre-dissected specimens) are more commonly used nowadays.

Attachment: The term given to clinical placements. The student is placed under the supervision and guidance of a hospital consultant and his/her team (firm) or a GP for a period in the course.

Biochemistry: The study of the structure and functioning of the body at the molecular level.

British Medical Association (BMA): The doctors' professional association and trade union providing representation and services for doctors and medical students.

BSc (Honours): *see* Intercalated degrees.

Clerking: Taking a history from and examining a patient on admission. A very useful learning experience if you are the first person to see the patient.

Computer-assisted learning (CAL): Computer programs are sometimes used to teach a topic in a more interactive format than a lecture/tutorial, and let the student set his/her own learning pace. They may also give the opportunity for self-assessment on a topic.

Consultant: The senior specialist doctor, usually based in a hospital.

Core curriculum: Under GMC directives the medical course is split into a core curriculum (in which all students must cover the same key topics to a high standard) and special-study modules (in which the student can go in his/her own direction and study an area of interest in more depth) which may not be covered by all students.

District General Hospital (DGH): A regional hospital, which treats a broad spectrum of patients, but refers more specialist cases to a teaching hospital. Medical students are taught by NHS staff, not university employed consultants and registrars.

Elective: A period (usually 6–12 weeks in the latter years of the course) when students can choose an area of interest to study independently outside their medical school, either in the UK or, more often, abroad.

Endocrinology: The study of the hormonal function of the body.

Epidemiology: The study of the pattern and causes of diseases in society.

Firm: *see* Attachment.

General Medical Council (GMC): All medical degree courses must be approved by the GMC. It is the medical profession's self-regulatory body, which ensures professional standards are maintained and patients are protected. Doctors must be registered with the GMC to practise in the UK.

Honours year: *see* Intercalated degrees.

Integrated courses: Integration is the merging of several disciplines into one (hopefully more meaningful) course. Integration may be partial, within a single year or phase (for example combining anatomy, physiology and biochemistry to teach body systems – respiratory, cardiovascular, reproduction, etc.), or it may be full, across all years, starting clinical teaching with basic medical sciences from the outset.

Intercalated degrees: Most schools offer students the opportunity to take an extra year (or two) in the middle of the course to study a subject of interest, leading to a BSc (Hons) or equivalent at the end. Some schools only offer this to high achievers, while others have an intercalated BSc (Hons) built into the course for everyone.

MBBS: The degree awarded to medical school graduates. (This varies slightly between schools, for example MBChB, MBBChir, but all are equivalent.)

Medical microbiology: The study of micro-organisms and the diseases they cause.

MEDLINE: A widely used and comprehensive computer database of articles published in medical journals.

Objective Structured Clinical Examination (OSCE): A relatively new form of assessment where the students are set several tasks: taking histories; examining patients; or performing tests/procedures to complete in front of the examiner within a set time. The student is marked according to a standardised marking scheme. Every student is thus assessed identically, ensuring fairness and comparability of results between individuals.

Pathology: The study of disease processes and their effect on the structure and function of the body.

Peripheral attachments: Placements in hospitals/general practices outside the university area and normally outside the university town.

Pharmacology: The study of the action of drugs and their application.

Physiology: The study of the functioning of body systems and tissues.

Pre-medical year: Students without the necessary science entrance qualifications can apply to do a pre-medical year which takes them to a sufficient level of scientific knowledge to join the medical course the following academic year (not offered at all schools).

Pre-registration house officer (PRHO): A newly qualified doctor working in the first year after graduation. House officers, while able to call themselves doctors and prescribe drugs, are provisionally registered by the GMC until they have completed this year satisfactorily. After this they achieve full registration.

Problem-based learning (PBL): Students learn from researching and solving a relevant (usually clinical) scenario, rather than being given all the information passively. Small group problem-solving tutorials, facilitated by members of staff, take the place of lectures.

Prosections: Pre-dissected cadaver specimens of the human body used to teach anatomy. These have replaced actual dissection by students themselves in many schools.

Registrar: A doctor who is undergoing specialist training (usually for between 3 and 9 years) before becoming a consultant or general practitioner. The next step up the ladder after SHO.

Self-directed learning: Learning under the student's own initiative from lists of objectives rather than didactic teaching (such as lectures).

Senior House Officer (SHO): A junior hospital doctor who has completed his/her year as house officer.

Special Study Modules (SSMs): Periods of the course when students study areas of interest outside the core curriculum (see above). These may be taught, or may be independent research projects.

Teaching hospitals: Normally the main hospital(s) in the university town or city. Services provided are part of the NHS, but the senior clinical staff will often be employed by the university and hold medical academic posts. Teaching hospitals usually handle specialist cases which can be referred to them from DGHs across the region. Many such hospitals will have regional centres for particular specialties or centres of excellence, such as cardiology, plastic surgery, neonatal intensive care, etc.

Viva: An oral examination (sometimes referred to as a viva voce).

Abbreviations

BMA:	British Medical Association
CAL:	Computer-assisted learning
CSYS:	Certificate of sixth-year study (Scottish students)
DGH:	District general hospital
GMC:	General Medical Council
OSCE:	Objective Structured Clinical Examination
PRHO:	Pre-registration house officer
SHO:	Senior house officer
SSM:	Special study module
UCAS:	Universities and Colleges Admissions Service

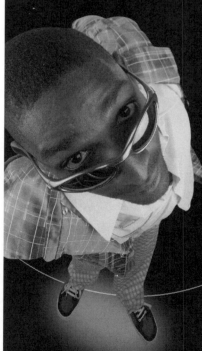